beautified

beau

Clarkson Potter/Publishers
New York

tified
kyan douglas

principal photography by henry leutwyler and ben fink

secrets for women to
look great and feel fabulous

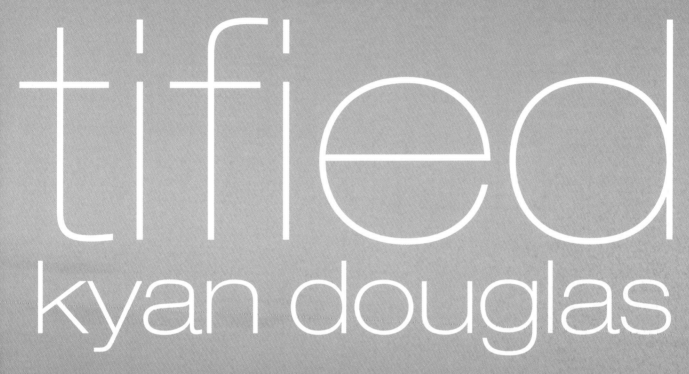
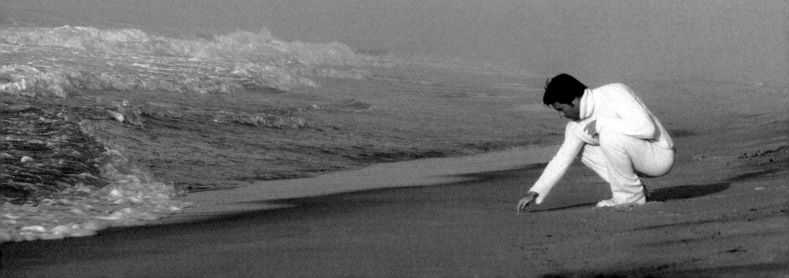

Published by Clarkson Potter/Publishers, New York, New York. Member of the Crown Publishing Group, a division of Random House, Inc.

www.clarksonpotter.com

CLARKSON N. POTTER is a trademark and POTTER and colophon are registered trademarks of Random House, Inc.

Printed in the United States of America

Design by Jan Derevjanik

Library of Congress Cataloging-in-Publication Data

Douglas, Kyan.

Beautified: Secrets for women to look great and feel fabulous / Kyan Douglas.   1. Beauty, Personal.   2. Women—Health and hygiene.   3. Hair—care and hygiene.   4. Skin—Care and hygiene.   5. Cosmetics.

I. Title.

RA778.D737   2004

646.7'042—dc22   2004016329

ISBN 1-4000-8144-0

10 9 8 7 6 5 4 3 2 1

First Edition

I WOULD LIKE TO DEDICATE THIS BOOK TO THE WOMEN IN MY LIFE: my grandmother, Mildred Virginia Goachee, who taught me to be true to myself; my truly beautiful mother, Judy Douglas, who has loved me without fault or condition my entire life, and from whom I get my spirit; and my amazing sister, Kelli Moore, whose strength, purity, and integrity I can scarcely find words to express. Thank you, ladies.

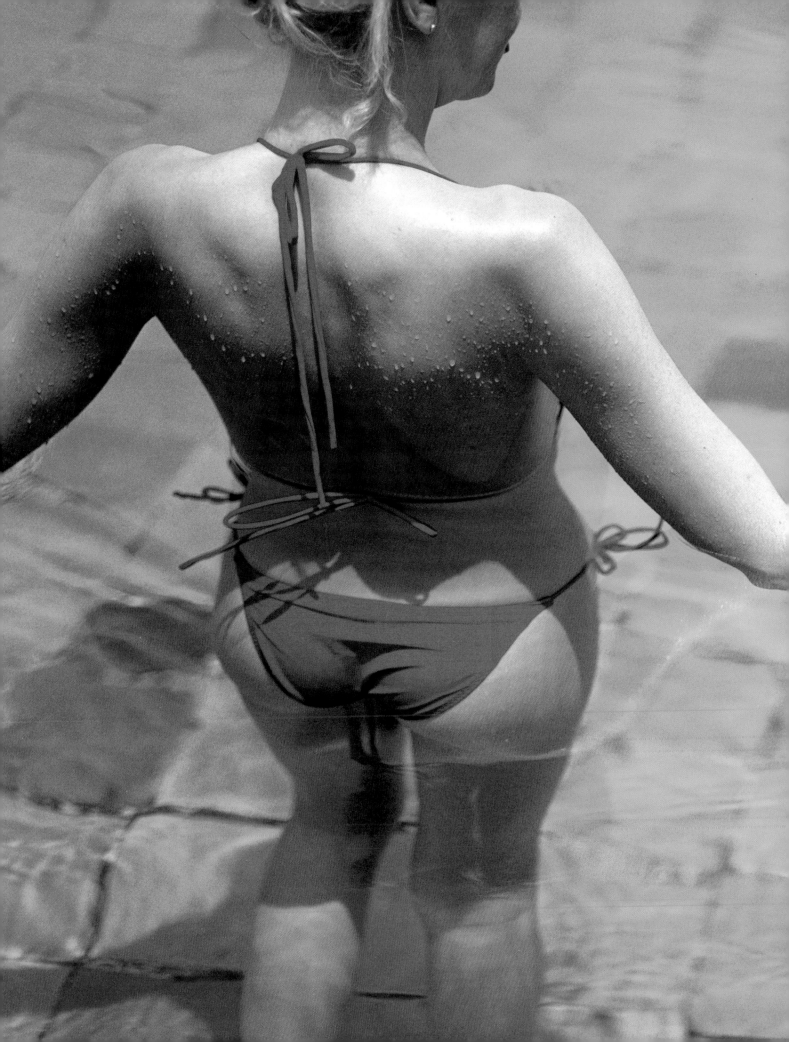

contents

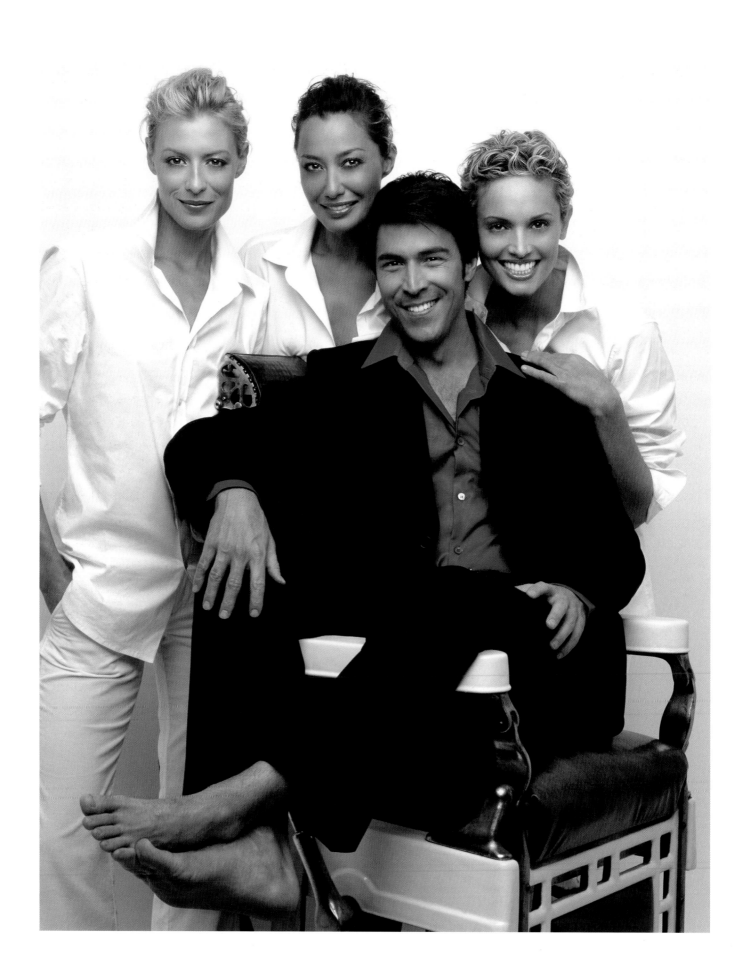

acknowledgments

There is so much to be grateful for and so many people to acknowledge for their contributions to this book and to my life. Because I cannot convey the depth of my gratitude, I hope that this simple thank you will suffice.

For their generous contributions in time, energy, and creativity that made this project possible, I would like to thank:

Kerry Diamond for her humor, passion, and commitment to me and this book.

Chris Pavone, Lauren Shakely, Jenny Frost, Doug Jones, Adina Steiman, Natalie Kaire, Marysarah Quinn, Jan Derevjanik, Mark McCauslin, Alison Forner, Tammy Blake, and the amazing team at Clarkson Potter. Also, Brian Lipson, Henry Leutwyler, Jeanne Newman, Ben Fink, and Chris Abramson.

A special thanks to the people who supported this project and me in ways I possibly will never fully understand:

Gregory Durham, my partner in every sense of the word; Michael Flutie, my manager and friend; Hilary Polk-Williams, my right-hand gal; Sean Ramsey; Eric Baptiste; Michael McConnell; Maurice Ettles; and Jenny Capitain.

And thank you to my brothers who I work with every day and whom I have grown to love and respect: Ted Allen, Carson Kressley, Thom Filicia, Jai Rodriguez.

I would also like to thank:

Ted Gibson, Nick Arrojo, Steven Margolin, Rudy Miles, Dr. Jennifer Salzer, Billy Yamaguchi, Calvin Klein, Kim Vernon, Jennifer Pinto, Ted Stafford, Vasoula Barbagiannis, Alexandra Schmidt, Andrea Leonarz, Julia Youssef, American Apparel, Kara Messina, Sephora, Origins, Borghese, Shu Uemura, Aveda, Tatami Mats, Hammacher Schlemmer, Scout Productions, and especially David Collins for creating *Queer Eye for the Straight Guy.*

Finally, I would like to thank the teachers in my life, past, present, and future. Some have guided me in the ways of spirit, some in the ways of grooming, all in the ways of beauty:

Ed Douglas, my father and the man I admire most; Perch Ducote, my spiritual brother; Dr. Diane Verdiano; Michael Ganther; Saxon Palmer; the Reverend Kay Hunter; Ken and Melba Ferdinand; the Jesuit Fathers at Loyola University New Orleans, especially Father Marvin Kitten; Mary, who showed me Inipi; Marianne Williamson; Kathy Zolzinski; Shannon Foreman; Erli Perez; Michael Smith; Cory Caballero; Thich Nhat Hanh; His Holiness the Dalai Lama; Swami Muktananda; Swami Chidvilasananda; Rabbi Michael Berg; Horst Rechelbacher; Annie Linden; Susan Miller; and all the teachers I haven't yet met.

introduction:
why beauty?

The simple answer is: because there's only one you. Why not be the absolute best version of yourself that you can be? I mean, this is it. This is your life and your moment. It is well worth your time and energy to be as self-expressed and happy and beautiful as you can possibly be.

I have a different definition of beauty than many people. I draw a distinction between being good-looking and being beautiful. Being good-looking is largely a function of genes, a purely superficial evaluation of one's physical appearance. Beauty is something altogether different. It certainly includes the physical, but it doesn't stop there. Beauty is the result of a quality of being, not the result of the arrangement of our physical characteristics. True beauty demands more than a great body or a cute face. It demands that we treat ourselves and others well. Beauty asks that we be kind, generous, forgiving, and gracious. Beauty insists that we develop our minds as well as our figures. Being beautiful is about cultivating our greatest intellectual and spiritual attributes in order to evolve into our very best selves. And, as a reward, those best selves will project our greatest physical potentials.

That is what I try to do week after week with the straight guys on *Queer Eye for the Straight Guy*. And that is what I want to help you with in this book. I want to guide you on your journey to becoming the person you are meant to become. A lot of the material in this book deals with tips and recommendations to help you improve your look. But the spirit of *Beautified* is about you being the best you can be in every way, not just physically.

In my own life I have gone to great lengths to learn as much as I can about "beauty" and "well-being." My goal was never simply to look good (although I wanted that, too). You see, when I was growing up I was extremely shy and felt painfully awkward. I just wasn't comfortable in my own skin. I made a decision as a teenager to change the way I thought about myself and to change the way I treated myself.

In my early twenties, I became deeply interested in my spirituality. I wanted to know who I was and what this life was all about. I made every effort to get to know myself. I did this through journaling and contemplation and through my education. As my self-worth grew, I became naturally interested in taking better care of myself. I began to work out, eat better, and think about my appearance as an extension of my self-expression. I became interested in the healing arts, especially massage. And before I knew it, I wasn't an awkward, insecure kid anymore. I was a young adult on a path of self-discovery who felt more confident. And looked it, too.

For me there has always been a natural synergy between improving myself physically and improving myself mentally, emotionally, and spiritually. That's why I wrote *Beautified,* to impart both practical advice and inspiration to any woman who genuinely wants to improve her life and feel great about how she looks and who she is.

In this book, I cover the basics on hair, skin, makeup, grooming, diet, exercise, and spirit. Most of what I discuss has to do with the physical you, the part that everyone can see, but your inner self is just as important. Mastering both realms is the key to becoming beautified.

As you know from seeing me in action on *Queer Eye,* my beauty rehab process involves finding the right products, habits, and regimens for each *individual.* I don't believe in one size fits all—not for makeup, not for skincare, not for diet, and especially not for clothes! My years of work in haircare and my studies in the healing arts have shown me that you can help people look and feel their best when you understand their lifestyle and personality. Then you can find the practices and tools that complement and enhance them without making them feel uncomfortable. Nothing's worse than leaving the hairdresser's or the cosmetic counter with a look you don't like or can never replicate. We've all been there and it's a drag.

Although the essentials of each beauty topic are included in this book, there are lots of tips and tricks for those well on their way to becoming beautified. I've included the techniques that were really helpful to me as a stylist, and things I've learned by testing hundreds of products for *Queer Eye.* You're also privy to the insider information I share with my girlfriends when they're having hair nightmares, breakouts, and other beauty dramas.

On *Queer Eye,* I've experienced the thrill that comes from helping someone identify the changes they can make to truly be their best. Sometimes the guys are unrecognizable with a clean shave, a new 'do, and a little manscaping; other times, the results are more subtle. Yet it never fails. No matter how drastic or slight the change, the guys are always shocked and thrilled. *Beautified* offers the same possibilities and promise to women. I hope you use it to find the courage you need to make a change, or as a source for answers to all the beauty questions you never thought to ask. There's nothing arrogant or vain about the pursuit of beauty—it's a noble cause, because the image you project to the world often reflects what people can't see—what's inside. It tells others that you care enough about yourself to put your best face forward. So let's get moving and get you on the road to becoming beautified.

a good hair day —
every day

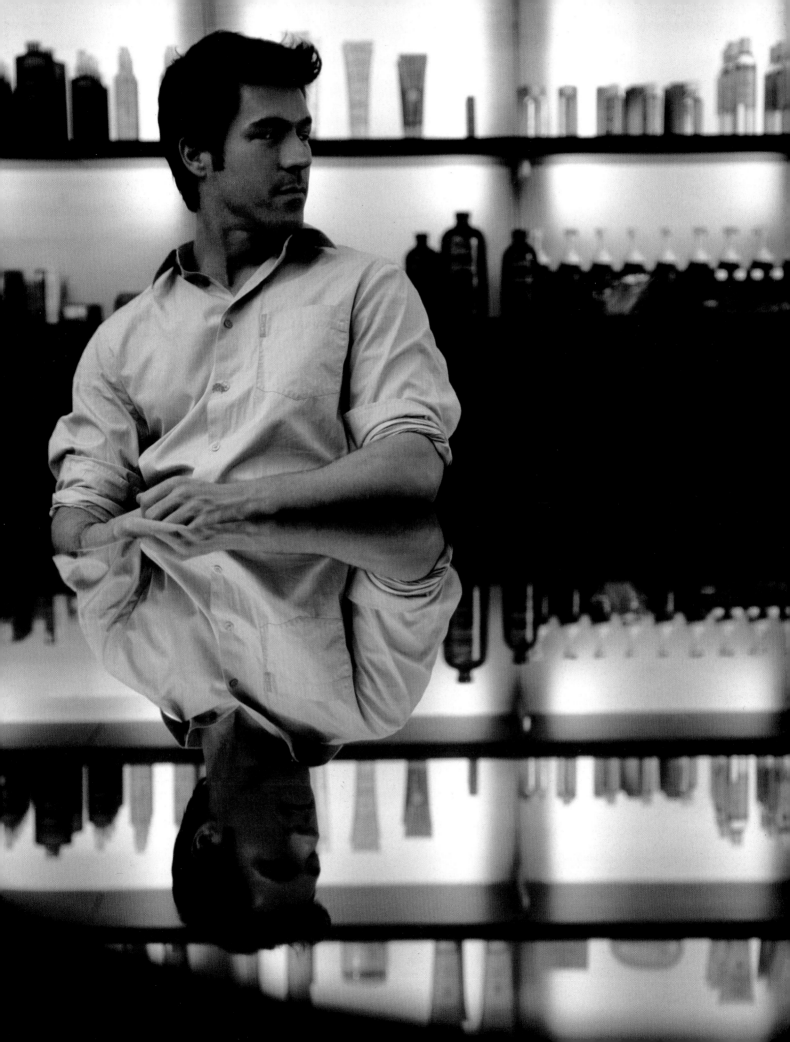

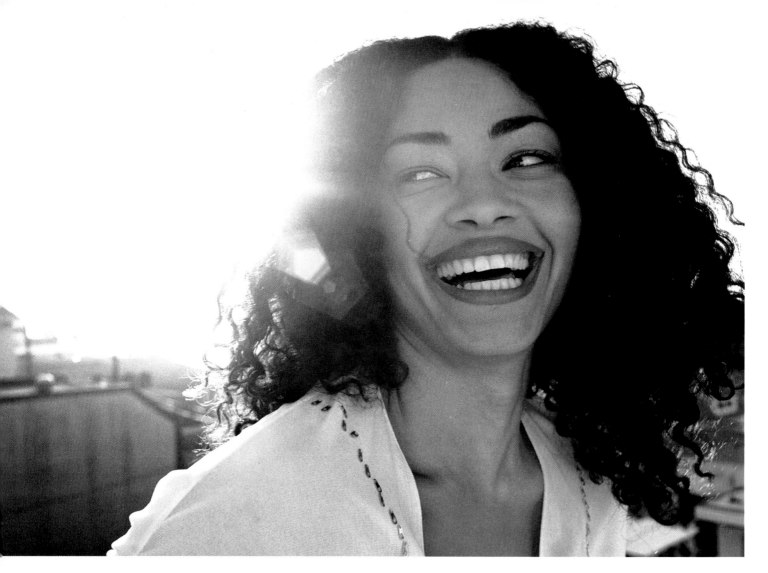

I can pinpoint the very moment of my hair awakening.

I must have been six or seven, and I was at my sister Kelli's softball game—
my parents had brought me along because they coached the team—when I
spotted this older guy with the most amazing hair. He looked just like Shaun
Cassidy, the actor and pop singer that everybody, including me, was in love
with at the time. I had an instant crush on the guy, all because of his perfectly
feathered hair, which was the complete opposite of the nerdy bowl cut my
father gave me every month or so. (My father was not a professional hairdresser; the only pro in the family was his sister, my aunt Helen, who owned a
beauty parlor.)

I remember thinking, "That guy has a very cool haircut. Mine is not a very
cool haircut. And I want to be like that guy." I told Kelli and she explained that if I
wanted feathered hair, I had to train it by blowing it dry and brushing it the same
way every day. Thank God for Kelli. She introduced me to the whole idea of
styling my hair and helped me realize that good hair isn't reserved for gorgeous
guys who look like hot actors. With a little effort, anybody could have good hair.

That's not to say I had great hair from the age of six on. I've had plenty of bad hair days, months, even years. Don't believe me? I've had perms; I even had a mullet. But through it all and through my training as a hairstylist and colorist in New York and my work on *Queer Eye,* I've finally learned how to get good hair. There's no magic involved, just some basic advice and a few tricks. Even I know, in looking back on my Shaun Cassidy experience, that hair is the perfect means of expressing your personality and taste in full force. Fabulous hair can boost your confidence, just as not-so-fabulous hair can make you shrink with uncertainty. Everyone deserves good hair, so let's get going.

kyan's good hair checklist

are you hiding behind your hair? Let the world see that face!

have you always had the same hairdo? Consider trying something new.

do you like your hairdresser? If the answer is no, find someone else. Getting your hair cut or styled should be fun.

how much time do you spend on your hair each morning? Half an hour? More? Life's too short for that. The right hairstyle can cut down on maintenance time and get you out the door much faster.

is your bathroom cluttered with tons of products and styling tools? You could be wasting your time and money, plus damaging your hair.

do you shampoo too much? You don't have to use shampoo to get your hair clean. Skip that step, rinse with water, and use conditioner only. Your hair will smell fresh and feel soft, and any protective oils will be preserved.

can't remember your last good hair day? It's time for a change.

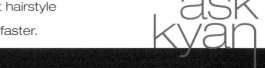

ask kyan

Q. How often should I wash my hair?
A. Not to gross you out, but I sometimes go two or three days without letting shampoo touch my hair. I just happen to like the way it looks when it's a bit dirty. If you've got oily hair or you work out a lot, you might want to shampoo as often as every day. The same goes for people with fine hair, because product build-up and natural oil can weigh it down. If your hair is weighed down with product buildup, but you have to shampoo it, skip the conditioner. That will give it a rest. If you've got chemically or color-treated hair, do not wash your hair every day. Every other day or so will suffice.

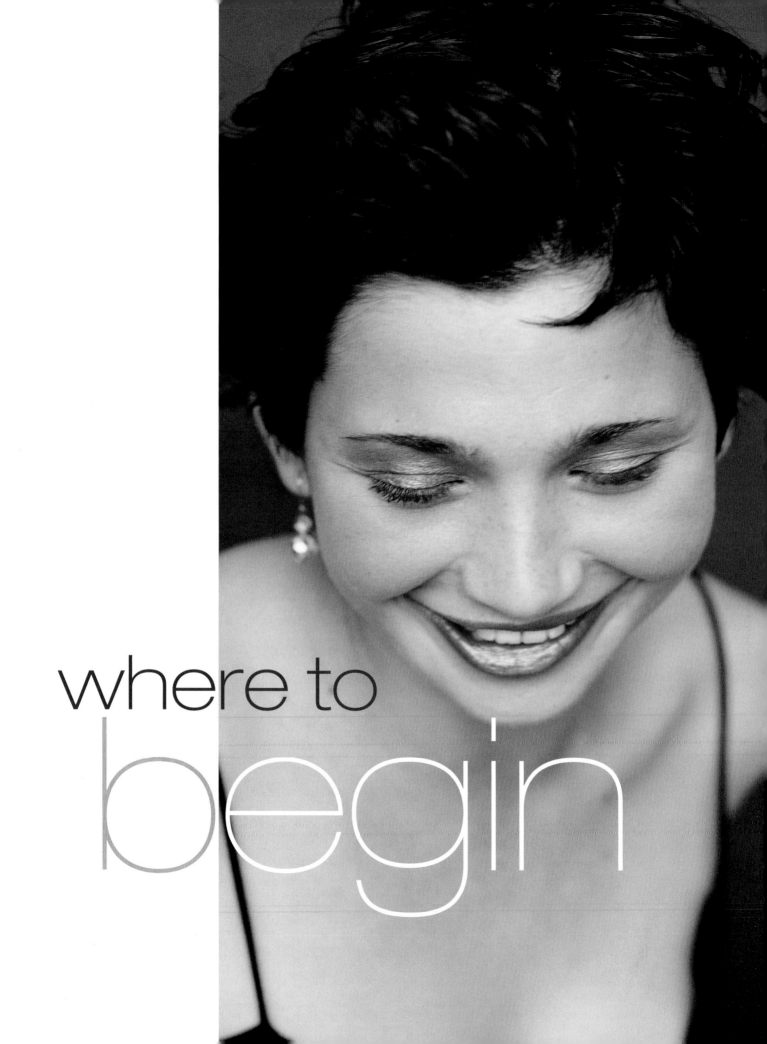

where to begin

Let's start with the definition of good hair. I love hair that flatters your face, has movement and shine, and begs to be touched. If you were born with great hair, thank your lucky stars and your gene pool. If you weren't, you need to start with your haircut. A good cut is the basis of good hair.

Signs that you've got a bad cut or that yours is past its expiration date? Your hair seems shapeless and/or too heavy, or you're making an effort, but you're never happy with the results. In other words, you're fighting your hair. And losing the battle.

the right cut for you

To get a great haircut, you need to understand what's best for your hair and your lifestyle.

short hair or pixie cuts require the most courage, since they'll take a long time to grow out if you're unhappy with the look. Pixie cuts are the shortest of the popular styles and are generally a few inches long (or less) when measured from the scalp. They're easy to maintain and are the quintessential "wash 'n' go" hairdo.

bobs are longer and fall somewhere between your ears and your shoulders. They're generally one length and blunt cut—no layers.

mid-length hair falls just below the shoulders. Its strength lies in the fact that it has the romance and ease of long hair but isn't weighed down as much.

long hair is great if you want to avoid frequent trips to the hairdresser and you want to be able to pull it back and run out the door when you're late for school or work.

When it comes to hair textures, make sure yours suits the look of your cut. Fine hair can look stringy when it's long, for example, and curly hair isn't ideal for bobs. Curls work better with layered looks.

Be realistic when planning your new 'do. If your hair is stick straight and thin, realize that a bob with a blunt cut probably won't create the most volume; you need layers, just like the girls with curls. Talk to your hairdresser about the cuts that are right for your hair type. Consider the amount of time and money that a new style will require, and think about what you're willing to invest. For some, getting up twenty minutes early to style is no problem, but for others, it's sacrificing too much shut-eye.

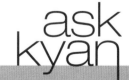

ask kyan

Q. Can I cut my own bangs?

A. There are so many questions in life and so few answers. But this isn't one of them. If you're an aspiring hairdresser, go for it. If not, put down the scissors and back away from the mirror. Most hairdressers will trim your bangs for free between your regular appointments. Ask about your salon's policy.

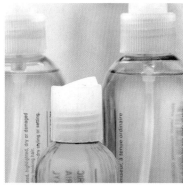

the hairdresser:
your best friend

Be honest. Do you love your hairdresser? Whether he or she is low-key and strictly business, wacky and gossipy, or somewhere in between, you should really like him or her. If your hairdresser is mean, bossy, inattentive, or worst of all, has bad hair, run!

The same goes for the salon itself. Do you like the vibe, the music, the décor, the receptionist? If not, it's time to move on. Need to seek out a new snipper? Ask someone with great hair for a recommendation.

ask
kyan

Q. How much do I tip my hairdresser?

A. The general rule is 15 to 20 percent of the bill. (The same goes for your colorist.) If your hairdresser owns the salon, they may not accept tips —ask if you're not sure. Don't forget the assistant who washed your hair. Anywhere from $2 to $5 should suffice, depending on the market you're in. If the assistant gave you a blowout, about $10 to $15 is great, depending on the market. And the coat checker? One dollar per item checked. Your generosity will come back to you in the form of excellent service—or good hair karma.

nick's mane advice

I've turned to my mentor, Nick Arrojo, for his advice on getting the perfect cut. Nick, who owns an amazing salon in downtown New York and is featured on *What Not to Wear*, has a wealth of knowledge about cutting and styling. He is a wonderful teacher, and these are some of his golden rules:

- **Don't get obsessed about what cut is right for your face shape.** It doesn't matter unless your shape is crystal clear.

- **Don't fight nature.** The further away you are from what's natural, the harder it will be to make your hair look good.

- **Determine if you've got a good cut or not.** How do you do that? Ask yourself two questions. One, did my cut last for a minimum of four weeks? Two, has anyone told me my hair looks great? If the answer is no to both questions, start looking for a new hairdresser or discuss the situation with your current stylist.

- **Length matters.** Anything below your shoulders won't change your face shape.

- **Don't wear your hair too long if it's fine.** You'll only play into the fineness. The longer it is, the thinner it will feel.

- **Don't go for a sharp,** one-length look if your hair is baby-fine because it will never hold the line. You want a feathered edge.

- **Avoid a center part.** You don't want a strong line on your scalp. Anything symmetrical will highlight the asymmetry in your face. Do an asymmetrical side part or a zigzag part.

- **Bangs will emphasize** particular elements of your face shape. But there are a few rules:

  If your bangs are too narrow, they will make your eyes look like they're close together.

  If your bangs aren't wide enough and long enough, your face will look narrow.

  If you have a round face, you want bangs that rise up at the outer corners of your eyes and that are a little longer in the middle. Don't give in to the natural inclination to cover up your cheekbones. The cheekbones accent the shape of a woman's face. Covering them up exposes the puffy part of the cheeks and the complementary contours become hidden. Highlight them instead.

  If you have a long, thin face and long hair, go for thick bangs, not wispy ones. You want to cover up skin and show a minimal amount of forehead.

  If you have curly hair, you can have bangs. Go for longer ones that caress your face and fall around your eyes to create more romance. Don't straighten your bangs and leave the rest of your hair curly. Mixing textures is the worst.

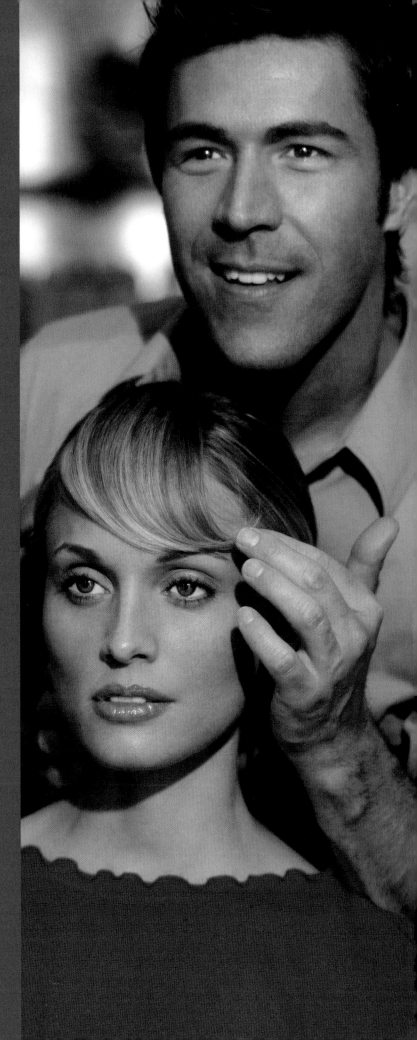

communication 101

Good hair is a two-way street. If you're not honest with your hairdresser and he or she doesn't dispense clear advice and recommendations, you'll never get the locks you're lusting after. Didn't like your last cut? Tell him or her why (be gentle) and discuss what you'd like this time around. Hairdressers are visual people, so make life easy on both of you and bring some pictures of actresses, models, whomever, with hair you love. Ask how realistic the look is for you and what it will take to achieve in terms of cut, color, and styling. The more specific you can be in terms of what you like or didn't like about your cut—or what you want from your new look—the more likely you'll get the results you desire.

When you're flipping through a magazine for pictures to bring to your hairdresser, look for ones from the red carpet, movie premieres, or personal appearances. Why? Those feature the most realistic hair you're going to find in a magazine. The star had a hairdresser come to his or her house or hotel room, got coiffed, hopped into their limo or electric car, and headed to the event. The hairdresser is not trailing the star on the red carpet, fixing every hair that's out of place.

Most magazine photos are taken at a photo shoot, where the model has a hairdresser plus an assistant or two hovering nearby at all times, using all sorts of tricks to make the hair look fabulous. We're talking wind machines, entire cans of hairspray, hairpieces, extensions, you name it. The photographer shines these incredibly flattering lights on the model's head to boost the color. Then comes the retouching, which magically makes the hair look even shinier, brighter, and fuller.

Bottom line—Not realistic.

Keep this in mind the next time you're wondering why your hair doesn't look like the lush locks in a magazine. But don't feel deceived. No one would buy a magazine filled with pictures of normal, boring hair.

Use other women as a guide to what you're looking for. If you're itching for a change and you find that you're constantly envious of women with a particular cut, and your hair type is similar, maybe that's the way to go. Pay attention to what you like and what you don't when it comes to styles worn by your friends, acquaintances, even women you see on the street.

kyanism

'Do Good Speaking of good hair karma . . . if you have really long hair and are contemplating a major change, consider donating your hair to Locks of Love, an amazing organization that makes hairpieces for children suffering from long-term medical hair loss. Don't let those beautiful strands end up on the salon floor—put them to good use. Check out locksoflove.org for more details.

color play

Once upon a time, when I was working as a colorist in New York, I couldn't look at anyone without doing a mental makeover of his or her hair color. These days, I'm not quite as judgmental about color. When I'm off duty, I'm off duty. But I still believe the right color can make a good haircut even better.

Trying a new color allows you to make a statement that will last for weeks, and even months, in just an hour or one afternoon. The right color allows you to complement your natural features in the best possible way, and it carries with it the freedom of trying something different without the major commitment that a new cut entails. The key to choosing a new color is to realize that you don't have to make a radical change. Some of the best colors I've seen on women are really close to the natural shade, and as a colorist I always urged women to try more subtle colors before taking a huge plunge—it allows you to grow into a new look if you're feeling the slightest bit hesitant. Subtle changes allow you to try new possibilities and be at ease with them at each step of the way, which is of course one of our goals in becoming beautified: feeling comfortable.

base color: Your natural color, or the color of the majority of your hair if you've dyed it

highlights: Pieces of hair lighter than your base color

lowlights: Pieces of hair darker than your base color

single process: One all-over color

double process: Bleaching your hair then depositing color (this is primarily done on blondes)

permanent: Color that never washes out

semipermanent: Color that gradually fades over time; can last up to twenty-eight shampoos, depending on the brand you use

toner/glaze: Semipermanent color used at the end of a salon color procedure to balance the overall tone

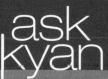

ask kyan

Q. My new hair color's too dark. What can I do?

A. If you or your colorist used a semipermanent shade, wash your hair with a clarifying shampoo or dishwashing detergent. Both will remove more pigment than ordinary shampoo. If it's permanent color, see a professional colorist. Whatever you do, don't immediately try a new color. The instructions on the box warn against messing with a new color right away, and they're right—trust me.

to dye for

Color is a simple yet super-effective way to change or update your look. You can go dark and dramatic, blond and beachy, red and racy, or you can try any combination of hot hues. I prefer natural-looking color that complements your eyes and skin tone, not color that looks like you're trying to fool everyone. But if you want edgy color, like platinum blond, jet black, or bold, chunky highlights, go for it. It's all about your personal preference and what will make you happy.

If you're a commitment-phobe, you can go the semipermanent route, or you can take the plunge and get permanent color. Then you need to decide between professional or do-it-yourself color. I'm biased toward salons, because I know the training that's involved in becoming a colorist and the expertise you gain working with color day after day. That said, millions of women color their own hair at home with good results.

But I want you to get *great* results, so read on.

salon smarts

Once you find your colorist, come prepared with photos to show him or her what you have in mind. Ask if your desired shade is realistic given your base color, or if you need to make some compromises. I can't stress how important this last part is. Having this conversation will save you from major disappointment and expense.

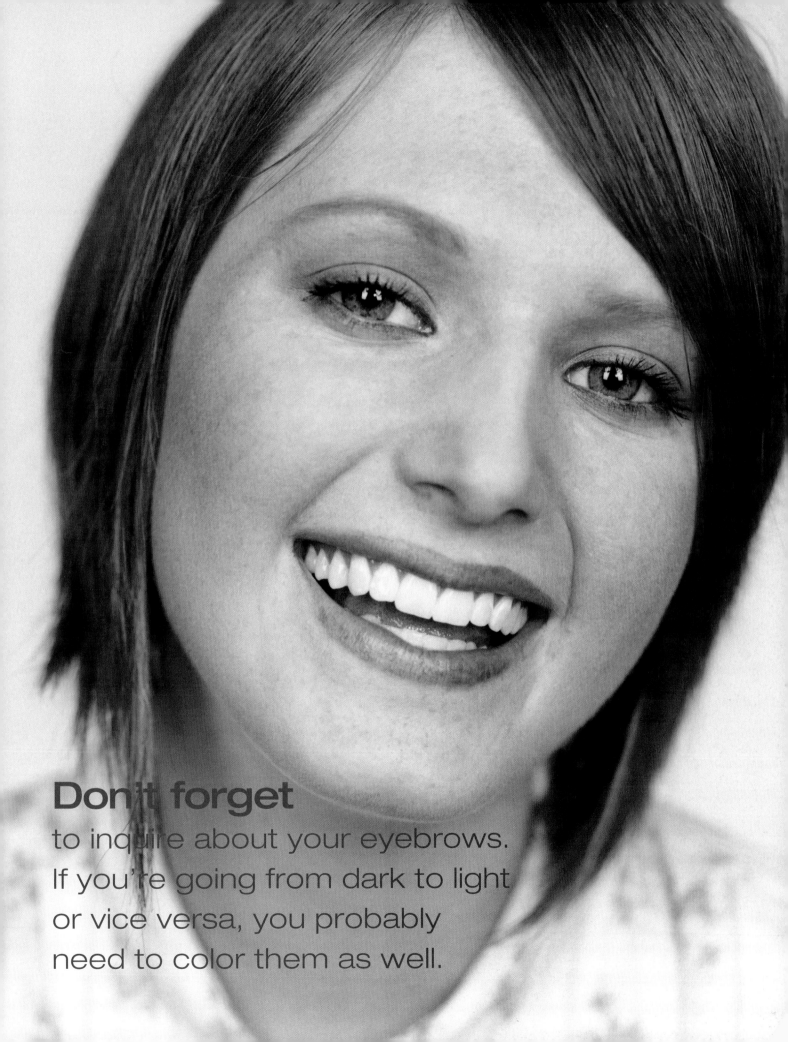

Don't forget
to inquire about your eyebrows.
If you're going from dark to light
or vice versa, you probably
need to color them as well.

adjustment period

Getting the right color is a process. Don't freak out if your new shade isn't what you anticipated. Call your colorist and explain what your concerns are. You might just need to swing by the salon and have your hair toned. It's not unusual to require a color adjustment, especially if you've gone from a dark color to a lighter shade or if you're working with the colorist for the first time. Most salons will tweak your color free of charge; just make sure you call right away.

Roots? Expect to get them touched up every eight weeks or so, sooner if your hair grows fast.

at-home how-to

pick the right shade. Don't be seduced by the picture on the box of the model with the great hair! Look at the color guide on the side of the box and make sure that formula is compatible with your existing color. What happens if you ignore this rule? You'll be disappointed. Again—be realistic with your expectations.

read the instructions. A lot of people ignore the directions, especially if they've colored their hair in the past. Do yourself a favor and check them out.

protect your clothes and your bathroom. Hair color can stain, so break out that ratty T-shirt and don't use your favorite white towels. Don't forget to cover the floor in case of spills and drips.

don't wash your hair beforehand. Unwashed hair is the way to go. The natural oils in dirty hair help protect your hair and scalp.

do a strand test. If you're new to coloring, or to a particular brand, follow the directions and test the color first. This way, you'll avoid surprises, tears, and a big salon repair bill later on. Buy two boxes of the same color. Use one for the strand test and the other for the full application (if you like the test results). Test a hidden section of hair at the nape of your neck.

watch the clock. Once mixed, the dye needs to be used immediately. Leaving on the formula for a longer or shorter period of time than recommended won't get you the results you want.

help! Most brands have a toll-free line and can explain how to correct mistakes or poor results. Check the box or the instructions for the number.

Color-enhancing shampoos won't boost the color of virgin hair.

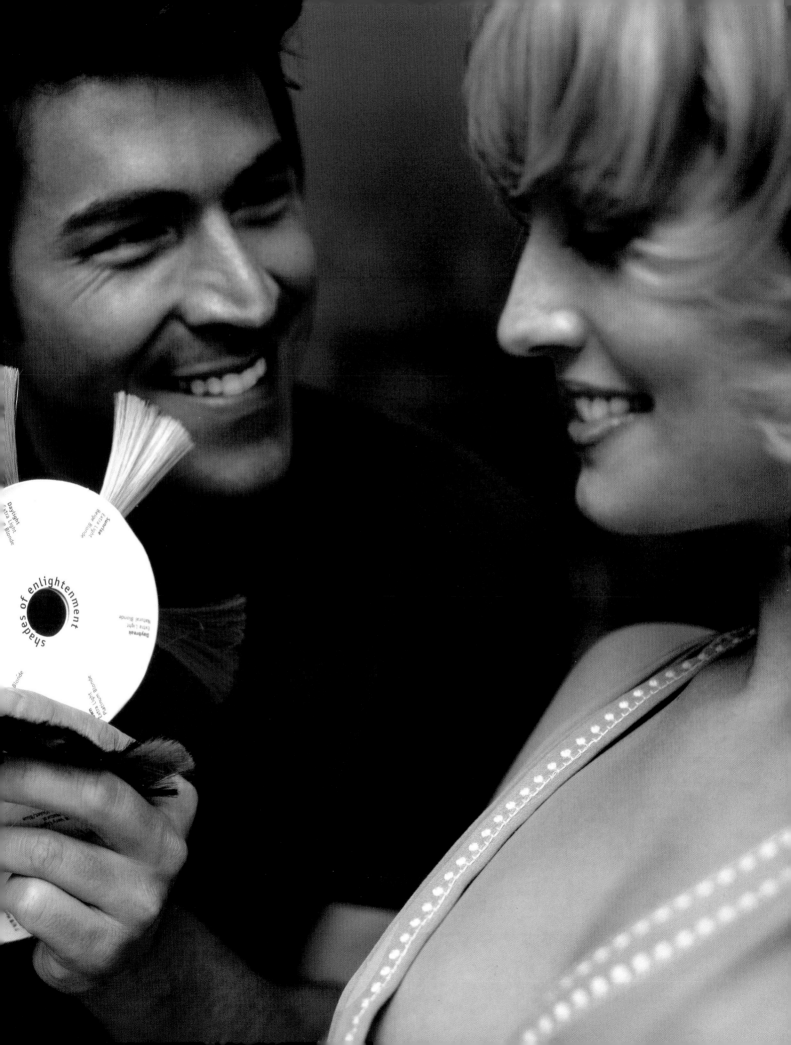

highlight lowdown

Imagine you escaped to the Caribbean for a magical month-long vacation. Now picture what your hair would look like at the end of your trip. I see pretty, sun-kissed streaks dappled throughout your base color. Most of us can't take off to the Caribbean for a month, but it is possible to acquire natural-looking highlights. It's a great way to perk up your hair without making a major commitment to color.

new hue, new you There are a few changes you need to make when you start coloring your hair. If we're talking about a radical shade shift, consider updating your makeup palette to something that's more complementary to your new color. You also should reevaluate your haircare products. Colored hair is more fragile than virgin hair and needs to be treated with T.L.C. Switch your shampoo and conditioner to formulas for colored hair and add a deep-conditioning treatment if you don't already use one. You can use styling products for color-treated hair, but it's not crucial.

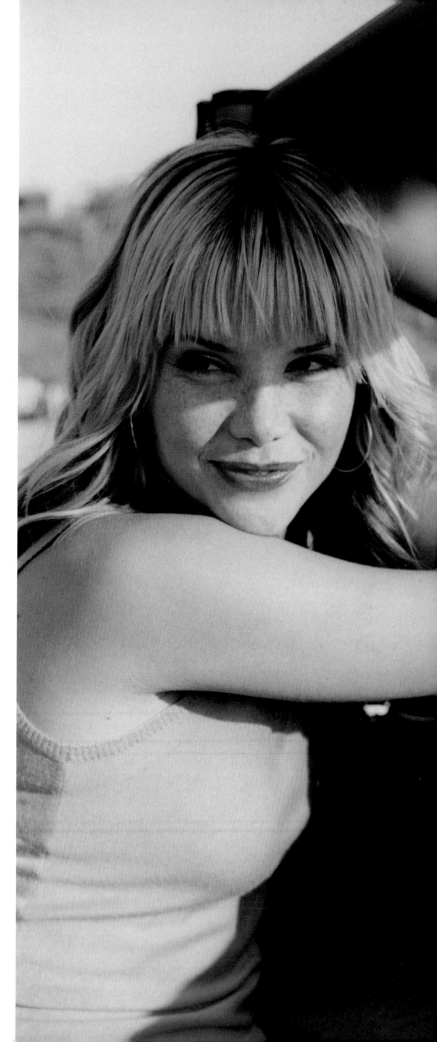

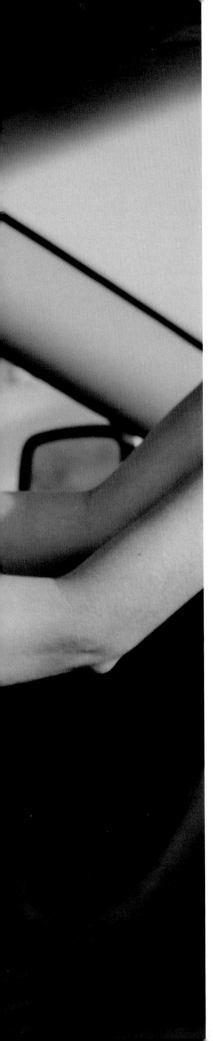

highlight how-to
Highlighting your own hair takes practice. For the best results, keep the words *precision, patience,* and *moderation* in mind, and follow these tips:

1. Don't rush.

2. Start on the right- or left-hand side of your part with the hair closest to your face.

3. Don't paint on the highlights in a clockwise fashion; if you do, you're bound to get very symmetrical, unnatural-looking results. Instead, do one highlight on the right, one highlight on the left. Don't line them up perfectly. The amount of space between each highlight should vary. Move right, left, right, left, from one side of your part to the other, toward the crown of your head, until you're done.

4. Don't feel like you need to do all your highlights in a single sitting. Try a few thin ones and see how you like them. You can always go back and add more or make the existing ones thicker.

soak up the sun
You definitely need to protect your color from chlorine and the sun, especially if you lighten your hair. A bathing cap's not the coolest thing in the world, but it's better than green hair—which is what you'll have after a few dips in the pool. As for the sun, there are plenty of protectant sprays and products on the market. You can try those, wear a hat, or both.

kyanism

D.I.Y.? Want to do your highlights yourself? As a professional colorist, it makes me nervous to think of people highlighting their own hair. It's trickier than single-process color, and it requires skill. However, the latest home highlight kits do make it easier than ever.

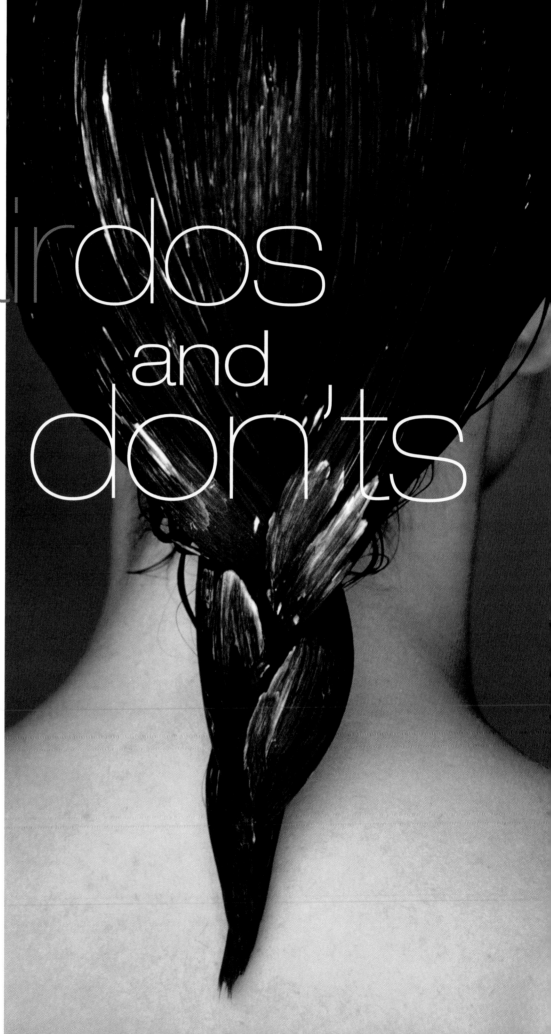

hairdos and don'ts

Be aware that you can't deep condition with an ordinary conditioner.

(Check the label to make sure your conditioner says "treatment" or "deep conditioner.")

obvious roots

If this is the look you're going for, fine. If not, you need to stay on top of your color maintenance. If you hate the constant upkeep involved in hiding your roots, maybe highlights are a better, less time-consuming option for you than all-over, single-process color. If your base color is light brown, dark blond, or lighter, talk to your colorist about giving you a "rooty" or beachy look. This involves weaving in lots of bright bits and making sure the color doesn't go right to the scalp. It will look more natural as it grows out.

two-toned hair

Whenever someone walks by with inches of dark roots, my heart breaks. If you've been coloring your hair and have since changed your mind, you have options besides growing it out—or cutting it off. If you're coloring your own hair, this is a great time to visit a colorist. He or she can closely match your ends to your roots with a semipermanent color. It won't match your roots exactly, and it will lighten over the course of several weeks, but it's better than that two-tone quality. You don't want to use permanent color because the lighter part of your hair will absorb too much color and won't match the color of your roots.

Another option is to add highlights, which will give your hair dimension and distract the eye from a less-than-perfect match. This should be done only if the difference between your root color and the rest of your hair isn't extremely different.

overprocessed locks

Does your hair look and feel like straw? Hay is for horses, not for you. If the color is too light, fried, and worn out, try a semipermanent color that's a shade and a half darker. This will give your hair some luster, restore a little dimension, and make it look more natural. Or you can get lowlights to help soften the color. If the color is fine, but you know that your hair feels very different from its natural state, read on.

Damaged hair is the result of good intentions gone wrong. Even if you've followed the color advice above, to restore damaged hair you must impose a moratorium on certain heat-styling tools and put away your blow dryers, flat irons, and other bad boys for a little while. If you absolutely have to use them, make sure to protect your hair with a thermal styling product.

I also want you to condition your hair like crazy. Look for a category of products known as reconstructors. These generally contain a protein that helps fortify the hair and actually rebuilds the hair structure. Start deep-conditioning your

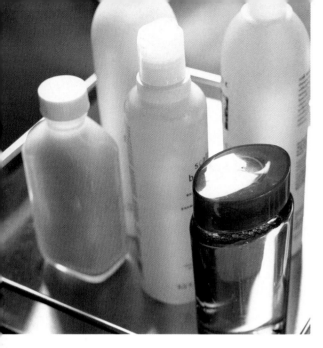

hair on a weekly basis. It's easy to do at home. Be aware that you can't deep condition with an ordinary conditioner. You need a product labeled specifically as a deep conditioner, reconstructor, or mask. Shampoo your hair first, then work the conditioner through, combing very gently from roots to end. I like to take a hand towel, soak it in water, ring it out, then throw it in the microwave for 20 seconds. Wrap your hair in that for at least 10 to 15 minutes to let the heat open the cuticle. Kick back and relax while the product does its job. When the time is up, rinse with lukewarm water and then cool water to close down the cuticle.

perms

These are a major don't, right? Wrong! While I certainly regret my own high school adventures in perming, every time I flip through a magazine and see some hot model with major body—hair, not physique—I'm tempted. Believe me, I understand that sometimes the perm calls and you must answer.

Although you probably will be more happy and satisfied in the long run if you find a way to work with the hair that God gave you, perms don't have to be a disaster. If you really want one, make the investment and find a hairdresser who specializes in chemical work. Not all hairdressers do. (When you're in beauty school, you don't do a lot of permanent waving. You just learn the basic patterns, which result in perms like the ones favored by old ladies with blue hair.) Talk to the hairdresser and ask if he or she uses different sizes of curlers (also called rods) and creative rod placement. Placing identical rods in a uniform pattern results in an unnatural-looking curl. Perm specialists, however, spend a lot of time developing special rod wrapping techniques and patterns to make permed hair look like naturally curly, tousled locks. Talk to the stylist about the effects a perm will have on your hair's shine and texture.

Remember: The word *perm* is short for *permanent*—and perms are exactly that. Don't risk at-home perms. If you don't like your results, you have no choice but to grow it out or cut it off—not a decision I want you to have to make.

ask kyan

Q. My hair is flat, straight, and lifeless. Is a perm the only way to get body and volume?

A. Not at all. You can try volumizing products, hot rollers, even the right blowout (you'll find more about these later in the chapter). Experiment with these options before committing to a perm.

crunchy hair

The only thing that you should crunch is your breakfast cereal—or your abs. When your hair gets this way, it's because of styling product. The main culprit is usually gel that's too thick and heavy for your hair type. Chances are you used too much or applied it to hair that was too wet.

crunch rehab is a two-step process:

1. rub a tiny bit of styling cream or pomade between your palms and start scrunching chunks of hair to break up the hard bits. Be gentle so you don't mess your 'do or cause frizz.

2. run, don't walk, to the store to buy some new styling products. There are lightweight mousses and gels on the market, or you can try one of the new gel-wax hybrids. Better yet, skip gel altogether and use styling cream or pomade.

P.S. If you let your hair air dry, some crunchiness is inevitable. Refer back to Step One.

If your hair is crunchy from extreme damage and not poor product selection, a haircut might be your only option. Hustle to your hairdresser, lose some length, and start over. Tell your friends I said nothing's chicer than short hair.

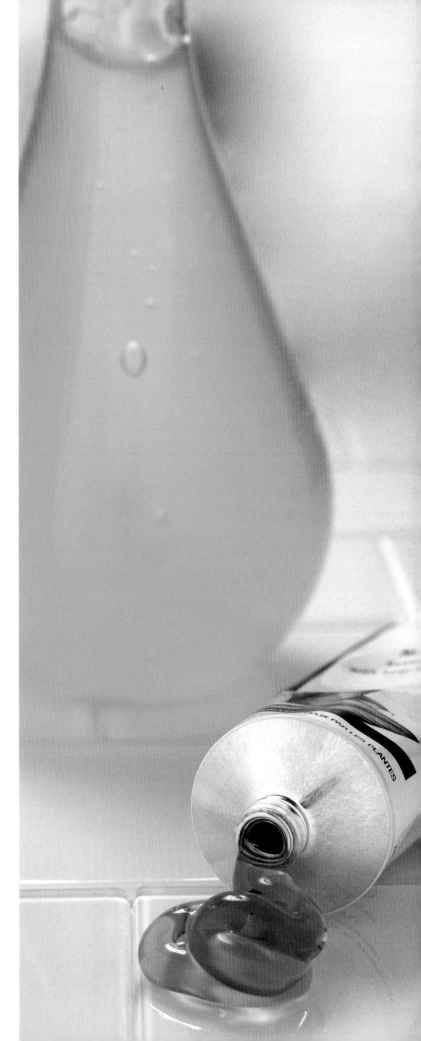

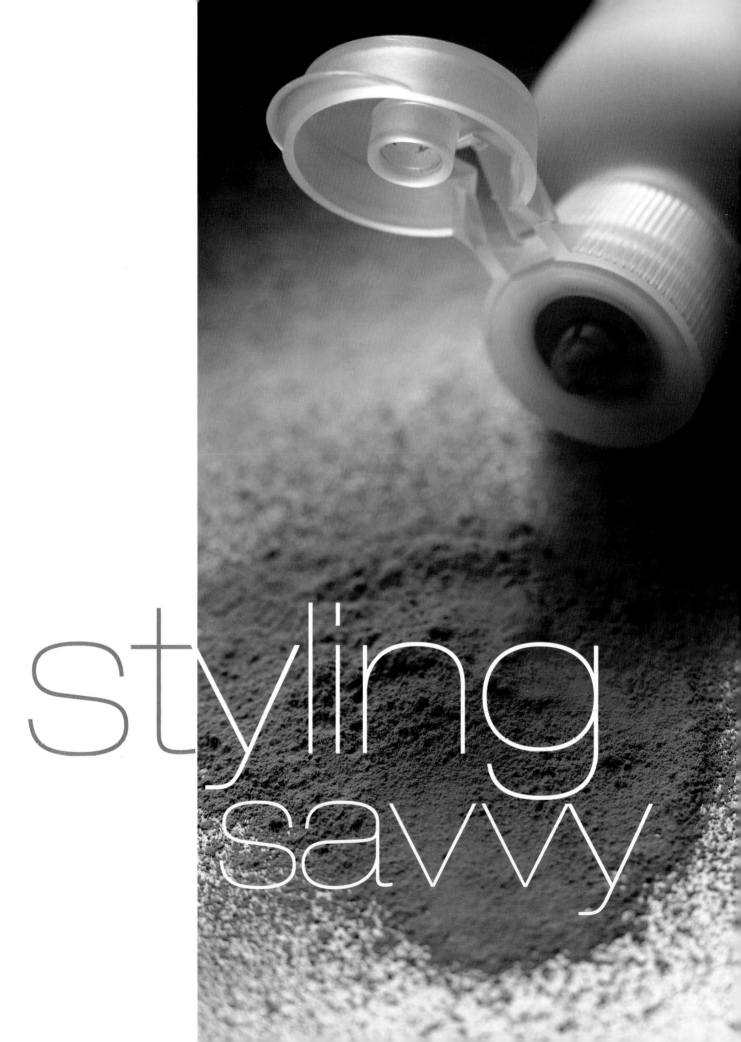

styling
savvy

Once you've got a great cut and worked out your hair color issues, it's time to style. Very few people have wash-and-go hair. Everybody needs a little tweaking, a little tszujing—or maybe a lot.

curls under control

Natural curls are gorgeous, but so many people with curls battle their hair every morning. They blow it out daily, pull it into a ponytail, or get it chemically straightened. Is this what you do? Well, don't fight your natural curls. Use the right products and styling techniques to keep them looking their best. Often, the problem is you don't know how to style your curls or you have the wrong cut. As far as the latter goes, the most important word for you is *layers.*

As for styling, some types of curls, like tight spirals, can look consistent day after day and can be controlled with a few spritzes of curl-enhancing spray or drops of silicone serum. Out-of-control curls take more work. Apply a bit of curl-enhancing cream or spray or light mousse, divide hair into sections, and twist each piece into a spiral. Let dry naturally or with a diffuser. You can leave the spirals in place or gently separate them with your finger and scrunch with a bit of finishing product.

curl caution

Don't mess with your curls too much after you add product and set them. Too much curl tszujing will result in frizzies. And layers are a must if you have curly hair, otherwise you'll be stuck with pyramid head, which doesn't look good on anyone.

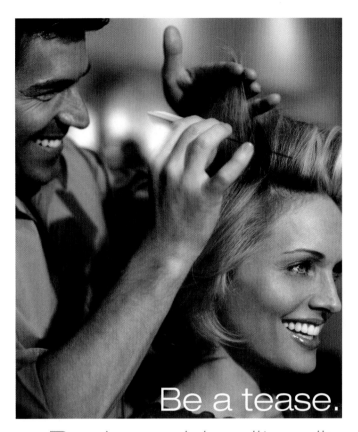

Be a tease.

Backcombing literally means combing toward the root instead of away from it.

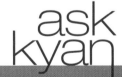

ask kyan

Q. What is Japanese hair straightening?

A. This is a heat and chemical process that gives you stick-straight hair. Some salons call it thermal or ionic straightening. It's a lifesaver for those with thick, unruly curls or frizz, but it's not for everyone. The treatment is very expensive and new growth needs to be touched up every three to six months. You probably shouldn't do this procedure if your hair has been chemically lightened.

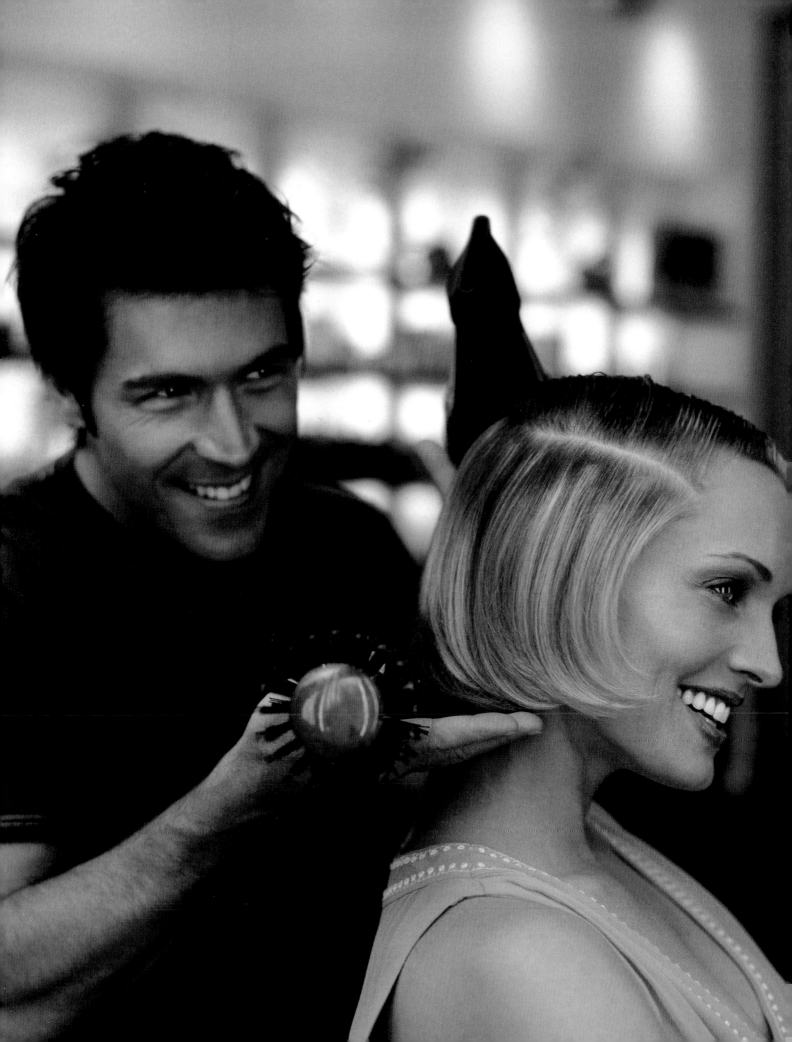

pump up the volume

Want fuller, sexier hair? A layered haircut will help. The longer your hair is, the more weight it has. Taking away length and weight via layers helps create volume.

You also can add volume during the styling process. You need a volumizing product, which causes the hair cuticle to expand and open up a bit, especially when used in conjunction with a blow dryer. Apply some product at the roots, use your fingers to create lift, and hit the hair with heat from your dryer. Pull the dryer away, but don't remove your fingers until the hair cools.

the perfect blowout

Love that chic, sleek look that only a blowout can produce? Whether your hair is curly or straight, a blowout will give you the control and finish that air-drying just won't. The key to doing it yourself is getting your hair as dry as possible before starting the blowout. If you're fighting and pulling your hair while it's wet, that's a lot of wasted energy. Towel-dry your hair, apply your product, and rough-dry with a blow dryer until 70 to 80 percent of the moisture is removed.

make your blowout last

1. **The less product you use, the longer your blowout will look fresh.**

2. **Sleep on a silk or satin pillowcase.** This is gentler on the hair than cotton and can prolong your hairdo.

3. **If your hair is a bit oily, but you don't want to wash it yet, try hair powder.** Light blondes can use baby powder. If your hair is darker, use a powder specially formulated for your color. Sprinkle a little on your hair, comb or brush through, and go. The powder is absorbed by the oils on your hair; it won't fall onto your shoulders unless you use too much.

4. **Is your hair looking limp? Backcomb it.** Gather the top layer of your hair and clip to the top of your head. Tease the exposed layer with a teasing comb (a special kind that has tightly spaced teeth and a long, thin tail). Undo the top layer and arrange over the teased hair. Instant volume.

kyanism

Stop the Abuse! If you're addicted to styling tools, make sure to use thermal protectant products. Give your hair a break from these tools every now and then and get rid of split ends with frequent trims. A weekly conditioning treatment is a must.

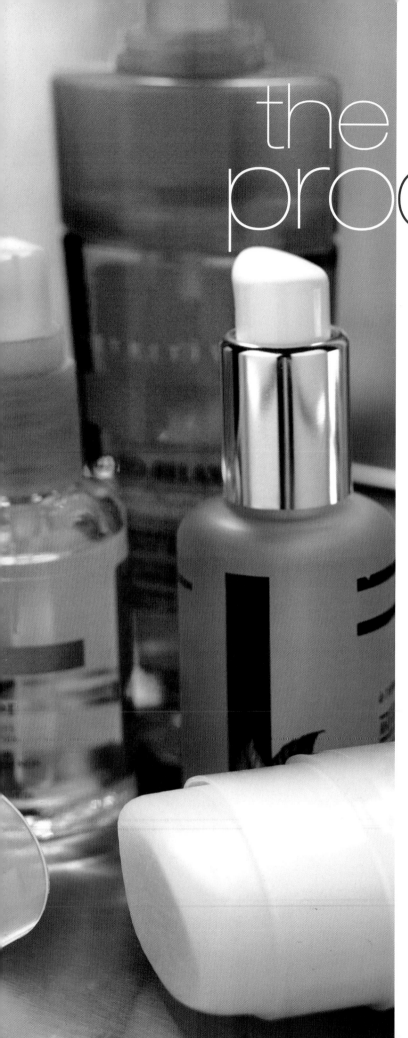

the product parade

It's easy to get confused by the massive amount of hair products available today. Whether you want to straighten, strengthen, curl, hold, finish, shine, protect, polish, or preserve, there's something out there for you.

gel This gives extra hold to any hair type. You'll find a tiny bit of gel makes most hair easier to style and more manageable. Heavy gels are good for slicking back hair (use sparingly); lighter gels are good when you want natural-looking locks with a bit of control.

mousse Great for curly and fine hair. Look for light formulas that won't weigh down hair.

wax Great on short, textured hair, or for keeping bangs swept over to the side. Use as a finishing product to give longer hair that piece-y look. A little goes a long way.

pomade This product adds luster and shine. It feels viscous and adds a bit of weight to the hair. Don't use too much or your hair will look greasy.

balm These tend to be lightweight and lotion-like in texture. Use as a finishing product or to control frizzies.

serum Usually a silicone-based product that tames frizz, enhances curl, and softens dry hair. Too much can make your hair look greasy.

hair spray Go for a lightweight formula. Don't spray the mist too close to your head or concentrate it in any one area; you'll end up with pieces that look stiff and shellacked. Best when used as an overall mist to keep your style in place.

too much of a good thing
The general rule with haircare products is to start with less, because you can always add more. This is especially true for products that add shine (use too much and your hair will look oily and flat). It's really about experimentation. Just because a pea-sized drop is perfect for me, it might not be the right amount for you.

On *Queer Eye,* I'm always telling guys to apply product starting at the back of the crown out to the ends of their hair, working toward the front. The same applies to you. If you start at the front, you'll get an overdeposit of product around your face. Distribute the product with your fingers or a wide-tooth comb. If your hair is longer, start at the ends, work up to the roots, and back down again.

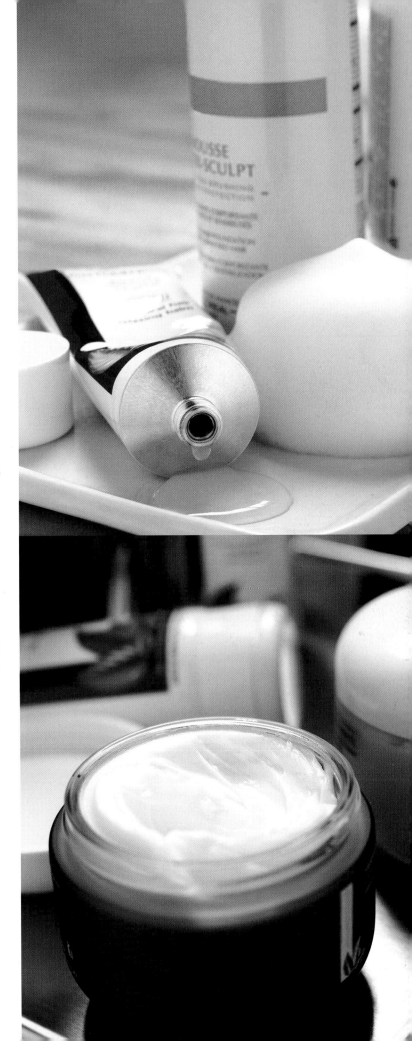

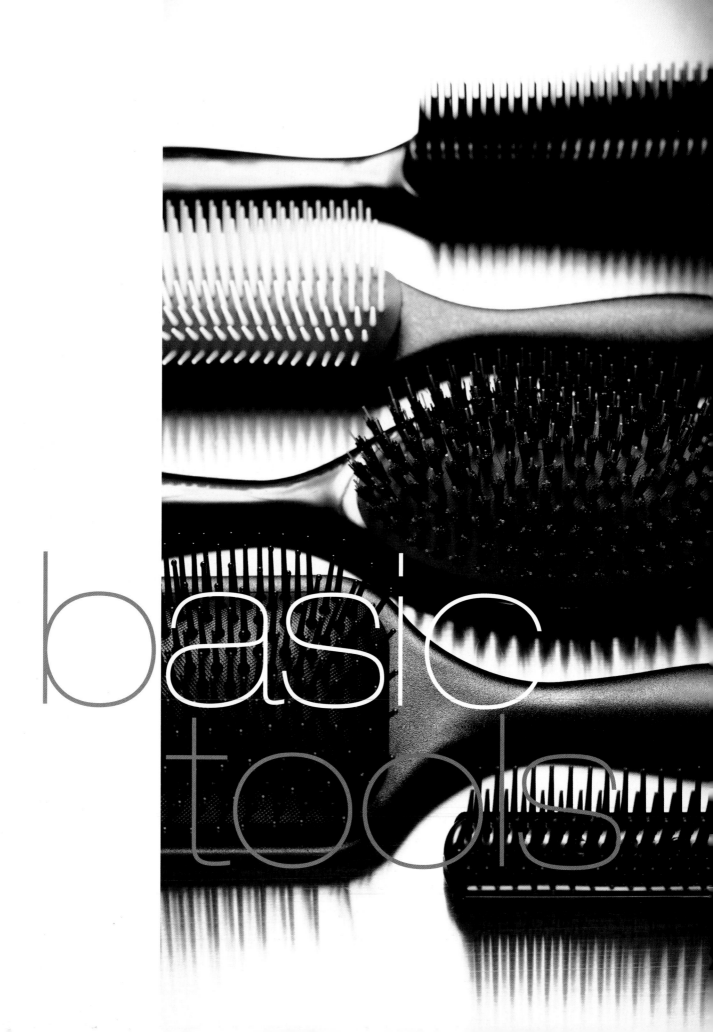

basic tools

brushes and combs

Everyone should have a good brush. Natural bristles, although expensive, are great for straight hair. If you have curly hair, you might prefer a brush with widely spaced plastic bristles. A wide-tooth comb is the way to go for distributing product through hair, and it should always be used when you get out of the shower. Brushing wet hair with a hair-brush will cause tearing and split ends.

paddlebrush

This is the best option for straight or slightly wavy locks. Divide your hair into small sections. Starting at the roots, secure one section with the brush. Keep an even tension and slowly brush from roots to ends. The nozzle of your blow dryer should follow the brush. (It shouldn't be pointed at your scalp.) When you get to the hair ends, pull the heat away, but keep the brush there—with a bit of tension still applied—and let the strands cool.

round brush

This is perfect for curly hair because you can get right at the root and maintain constant tension, and it's an option for straight hair because it allows you to curl the ends and lift the hair at the root, which creates more volume. Follow the same instructions as above, but don't wrap the hair around the brush, unless you want the ends to flip in or out. When you get to the hair ends, make sure to twirl the brush for the desired curl.

clean freak

Make sure to wash your brushes and combs with soap and warm water every week or so. Let air dry. Brushes and combs get pretty gross when they're caked with dust, hair, and product residue. Remember to remove the strands of hair from them after each use.

hair dryers

Great ones are available at every price point. You don't need an expensive professional model unless you're an actual professional or you do your own blowouts. I recommend getting an 1,800-watt model, if not higher.

If you have curly hair, buy a diffuser attachment. This literally diffuses the heat around your head, which is better than isolated, concentrated bursts. It makes for an easier styling experience and will keep your hair healthy, preserve your curls, and cut down on frizz.

kyanism

Take It Easy When I say tension, I don't mean a kung fu grip. Don't be so rough that you're tugging or pulling at your hair. Make sure you have a nozzle attachment for your blow dryer. This allows you to focus the hot air directly on the brush, where you're applying the tension.

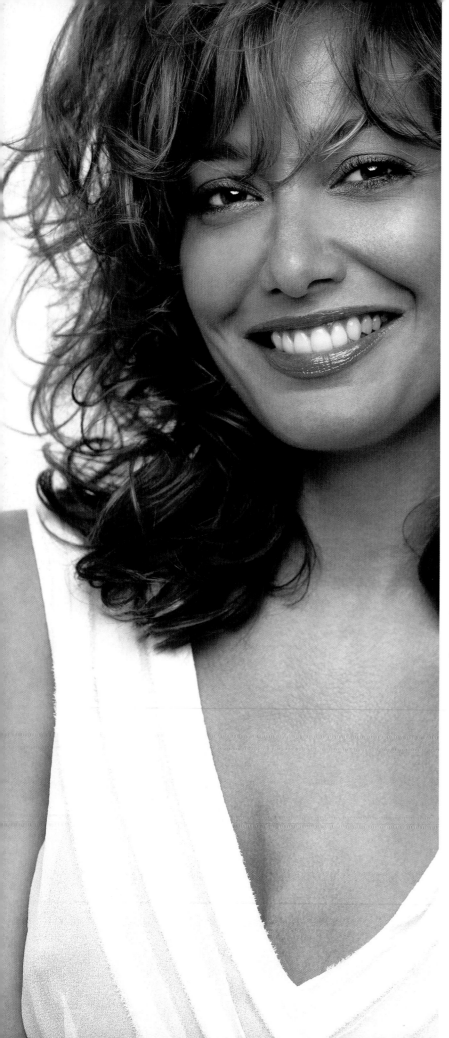

curling and straightening irons

These are terrific when you're doing your hair for a special event. If you're using them every day, though, you could be doing real damage.

hot rollers

An easy way to add volume and curl. Don't put piping-hot rollers in your hair. Let them cool a bit. Once you've put them in your hair, let them cool completely before removing. Jumbo rollers will result in loose curls; small ones in tighter curls.

Experiment with how you wind the hair around the roller or the barrel. Winding it horizontally (parallel to the floor) will result in more curl at the hair ends. Try winding rollers vertically for a more spiraled, tousled look.

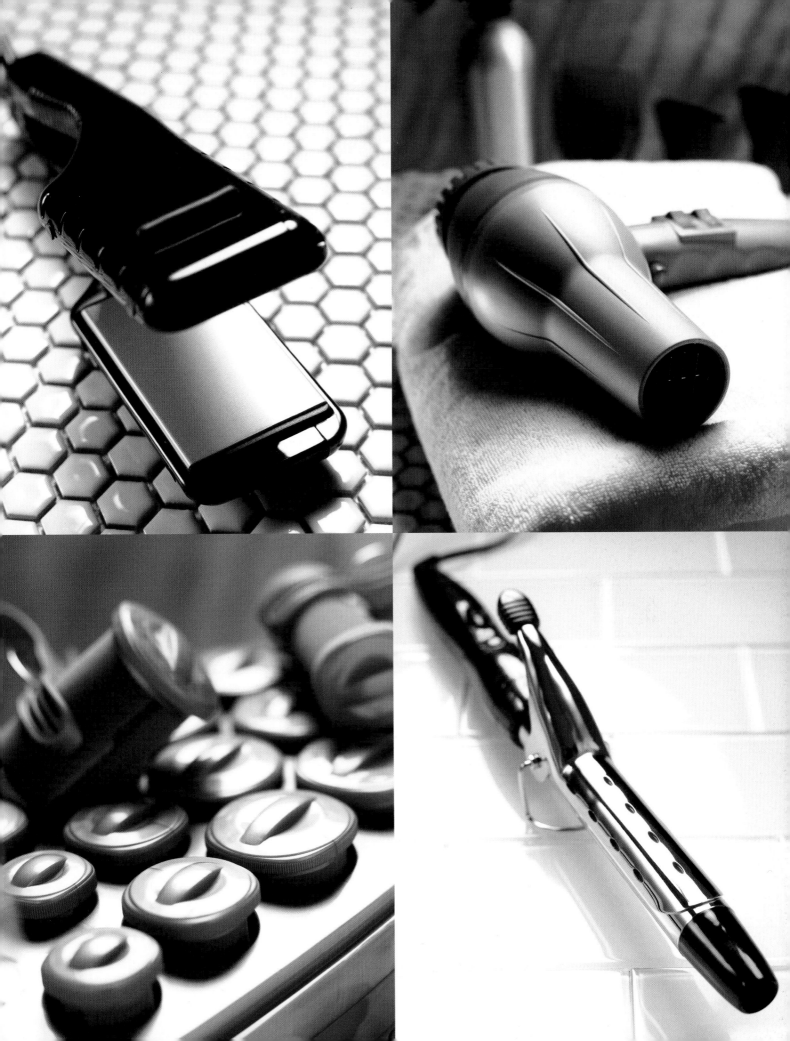

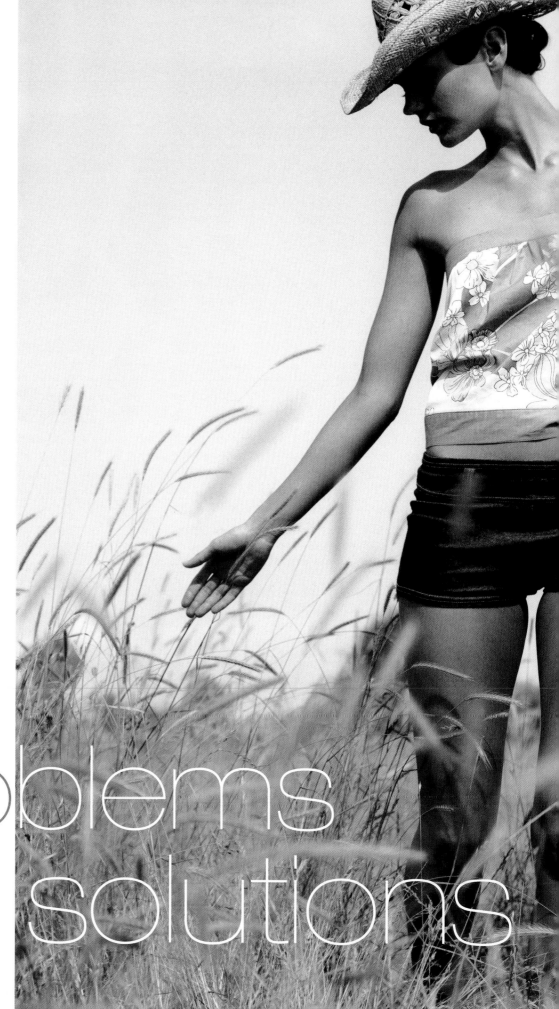

problems
& solutions

flaky personality? Don't be embarrassed if you have dandruff. It has various causes, many of which are hard to control, like heredity, stress, and allergies. Try an over-the-counter dandruff shampoo and make sure to follow the directions. If that fails, see a dermatologist. He or she can prescribe a stronger shampoo or topical product. But don't rely on medicine alone. If you have dandruff, take a look at your lifestyle, diet, and stress level and make some positive changes. Such things as drinking alcohol, smoking, and dehydration often exacerbate skin problems.

hair loss This is nothing to be ashamed of. It's not as common for women to lose their hair as it is for men, but it still happens and it can be depressing and distressing when it does. If you notice an abnormal amount of hair loss or any bald patches, call a dermatologist. He or she can determine the problem and prescribe medication or an over-the-counter solution. Discuss your diet, lifestyle, and stress level with your doctor, because those factors could be contributing to the problem.

emergency style solutions

not

not The baseball cap is the classic response to bad hair, but it's a lazy option.

not Banana clips are one of the very few things in life that I categorically dislike. Toss your banana clips!

not Bandannas can look cool—sometimes. But they also can give off that unwashed hippy vibe. Use sparingly. Save your bandannas for the beach and for weekends.

hot

hot Any other hat—fedoras, cowboy hats, newsboy caps, skullcaps—can be really stylish

hot Other hair accessories can be chic. Headbands, ponytail wraps, and barrettes are a much more stylish option.

hot Headscarves are a better option. I'd rather see a great scarf folded into a triangle and tied around your head. Try a plain black one or a brightly printed one. Silk scarves are dressier, but can slip off your hair; cotton has more staying power.

kyanism

Bad Hair Minutes
I really dislike the term "bad hair day." It implies that an entire day is ruined because you're unhappy with your hair. We've all been there and we've all realized that life goes on, despite a temporarily dreadful 'do. I prefer to have a "bad hair minute," which is basically the moment you realize you're not loving your hair, acknowledge the situation, devise a solution, and then move on. You'll save the day.

beauty is skin deep

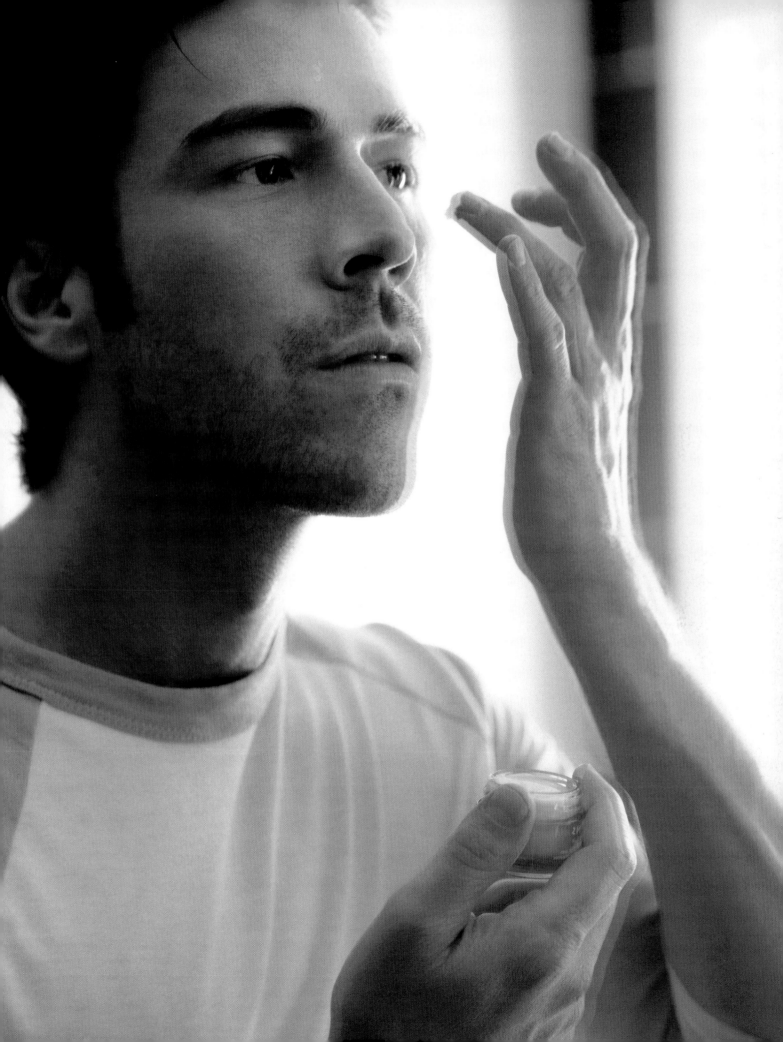

Most children don't get into skincare, but I've been obsessed since grammar school. Back then, my mother Judy had a vanity table in her bedroom covered with more creams and lotions than you can imagine, and I always thought there was something magical about them. Almost every day, I'd watch her go through her routine, and when she was out of sight, I'd slather her products all over my face. Believe me, I had the softest skin of any kid on the block.

I'm lucky I had a mother who was so forward thinking about skincare. She had a solid regimen, and she even had a dermatologist before that was a common thing to do. Clearly, her fastidiousness about her face rubbed off on me. Today, my version of her vanity table is the medicine cabinet in my bathroom. It's filled with face scrubs, eye creams, cleansers, sunscreens, and, of course, my favorite product, moisturizer. (Confession: I probably have 30 different moisturizers in my apartment right now.) Like I told you, I'm obsessed.

Every week, I try dozens of new items and road-test new procedures, from body peels to electrostimulation facials, to find the perfect grooming solutions for the *Queer Eye* straight guys. But you know what? I enjoy it so much that I'd do it even if it wasn't a true "responsibility." I really believe that good skin is worth taking the time and effort to achieve. A radiant complexion makes you feel great and it certainly boosts your confidence. Your skin is what people see on the outside, but it is often an accurate reflection of what's going on inside—of the food you put into your body, of the water you drink, of your stress levels. Your skin reveals all of this. Beautified skincare means that you're taking care of your skin by keeping these components in check. But it also means using the right treatments and products, and following the right routines to keep your skin in top shape. These are the guidelines that are covered in this chapter. It's my goal to help you put your best face forward, so let's get going.

what's your type?

Tall, slim, blond? Wait, we're talking about your skin, not potential boyfriends. Once you know your skin type, you can craft the perfect skincare routine.

normal • Your skin is neither too dry nor too oily.

dry • Your skin feels tight after you wash it. You might have dry or flaky patches.

oily • Your skin is shiny and sometimes oily to the touch.

combination • Your nose and perhaps forehead and chin (your T-zone) are oily. Your cheeks and under-eye area are dry or normal.

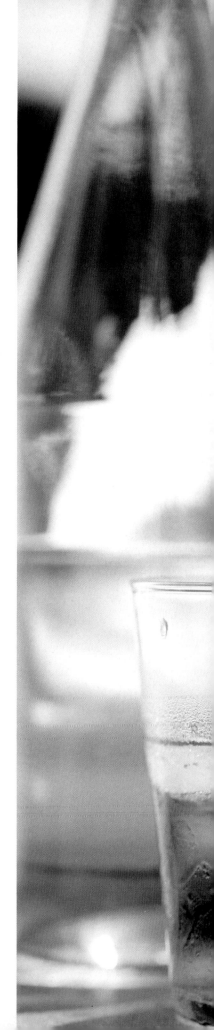

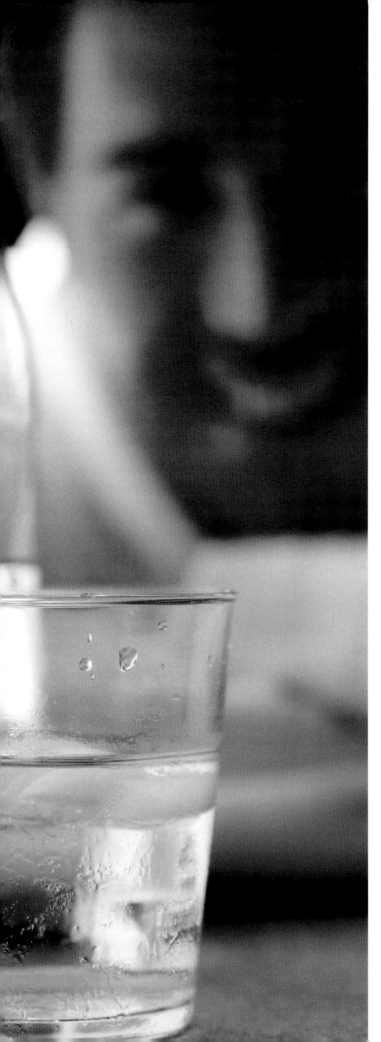

kyan's smart
skin strategies

don't let your skin stress you out.
Trust me. You can improve your complexion, no matter how bad it is.

stick to a routine. Commit yourself to a regimen that you follow day and night. Consistency is key.

show your skin some love. It's not enough to use the right products on your skin. Many other factors contribute to your complexion, so you also must follow these rules:

> drink enough water.
> eat well.
> get enough sleep.
> limit your sun exposure.
> don't smoke.
> control your stress level.

I know lots of people with bad habits who have perfect skin. They eat tons of junk food and go to bed every night with their makeup on, yet they never get a pimple. Life's unfair that way, but don't dwell on it. Take action.

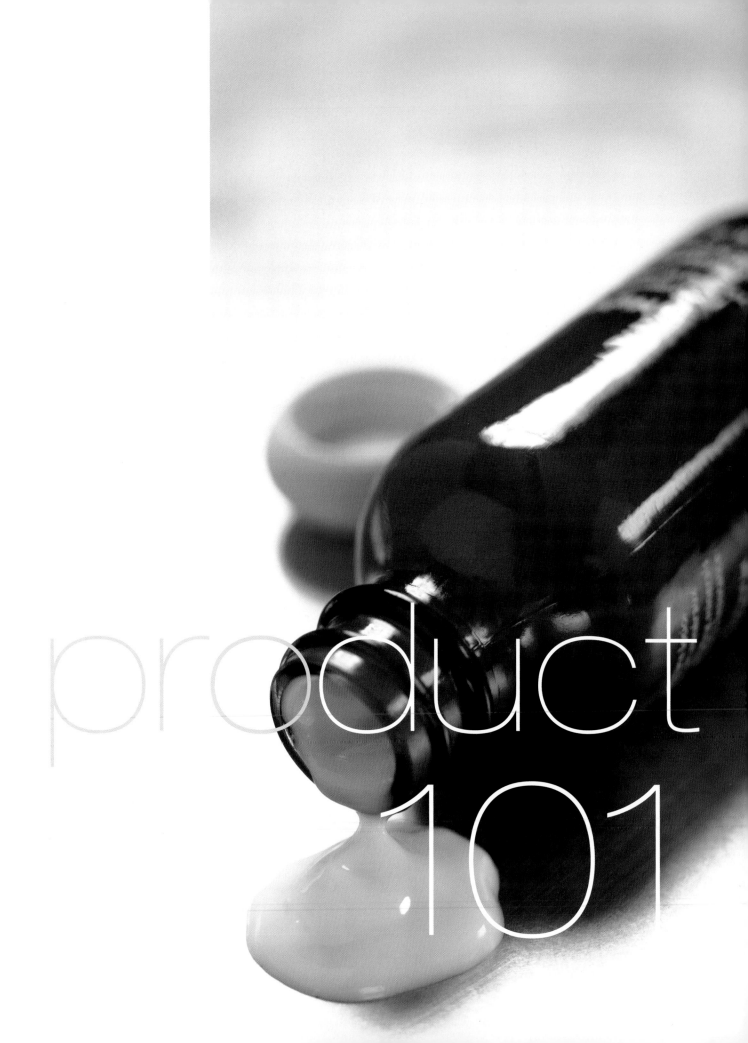

product
101

before we get to the skincare routine that's right for you, let's consider the different products out there.

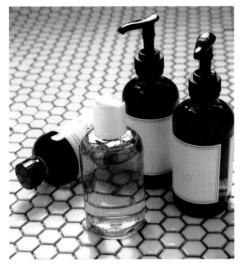

cleanser
Removes the grime of the day, makeup, oil, dead skin cells, and more. Certain cleansers contain additional ingredients to fight acne, wrinkles, or dull skin.

foaming cleansers
Best for oily and combination skin types.

creamy cleansers
Best for dry skin. Some creamy cleansers foam up, however. If you have dry skin, be sure to use the non-foamy kind.

cleansing cloths
These are towelettes that cleanse, remove makeup, and/or exfoliate. I only recommend them for taking off makeup. They're not a replacement for a good cleansing regimen.

toner
These light liquid solutions hydrate, remove any traces of grime or cleanser left behind after you've washed your face, and prime your skin for moisturizer. You can use a toner that has ingredients to fight acne or wrinkles, or one that helps balance dry or oily skin.

kyanism
Tone It Down! Do not use a toner that strips your skin of essential oils. If your face feels squeaky clean afterward, your toner is too strong. Since it removes all the emollients and oils from your skin, your body might overcompensate by producing too much oil. Skin should feel moist and refreshed after using toner, not dry and tingly.

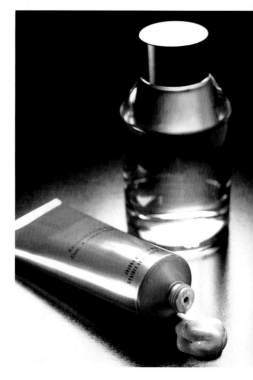

Es·the·ti·cian *(n)* A person who performs beauty treatments at a spa, salon, or doctor's office.

exfoliant I'm on a mission to get

the world to exfoliate, especially the straight guys we help on the show. So many of them are exfoliating virgins, but I'm sure you're savvy about scrub. Exfoliation makes everyone's skin look better because you're removing dead skin cells to reveal the brighter, fresher skin underneath.

manual exfoliant These are scrubs that rub away

dead skin. Key ingredients can include oatmeal, ground-up apricot kernels, walnut shells, or superfine crushed marble.

A new kind of manual exfoliant is the micro-dermabrasion scrub. At a micro-dermabrasion procedure, your skin is gently sandblasted with millions of tiny aluminum oxide crystals. The doctor or esthetician uses a machine that sprays these crystals directly onto your skin. Micro-dermabrasion feels like the slightly sandpaper-ish feel of a cat's tongue. The result? Super-smooth skin.

Today, beauty brands are taking those very same aluminum oxide crystals and putting them into manual scrubs for at-home usage. I don't find these to be any better or worse than other scrubs on the market; the main difference is in the feel, because the crystals are extremely fine. These crystals are the finest of all available scrubs, so they feel softer on the skin.

chemical exfoliant These are acids that speed the

exfoliation process and enhance cell renewal. The two most common in beauty products are alpha hydroxy acids, or AHAs (glycolic acid is one example), and beta hydroxy acids, or BHAs (such as lactic and salicylic

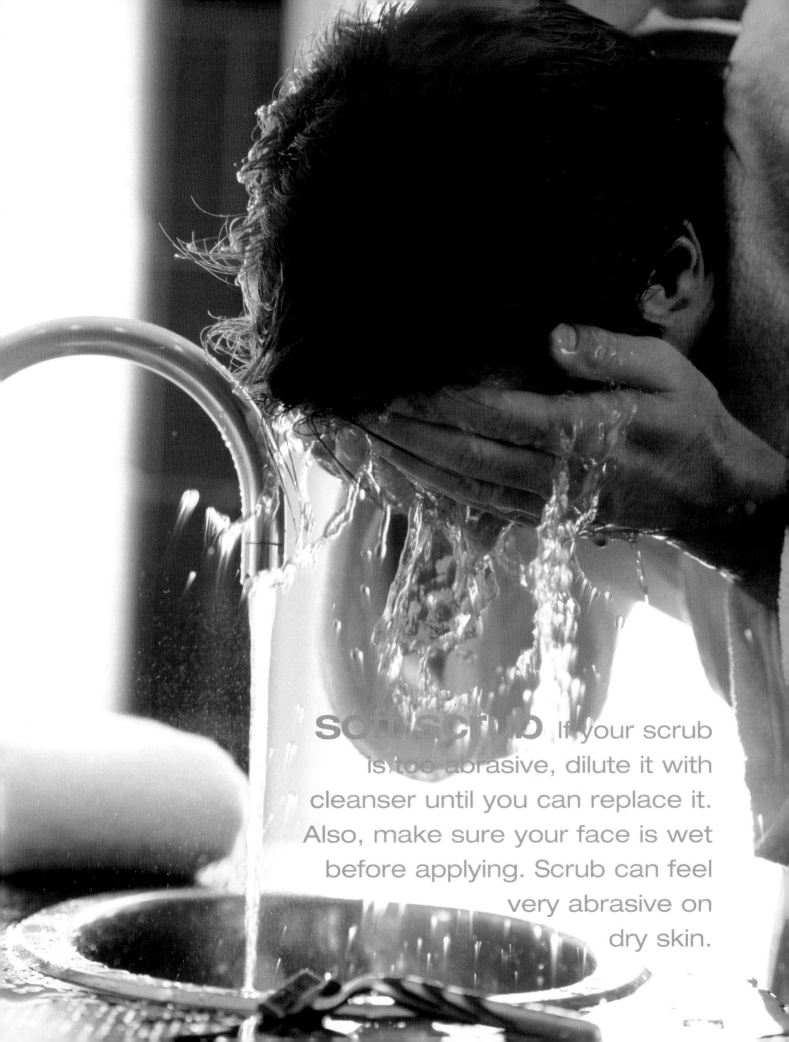

softscrub If your scrub is too abrasive, dilute it with cleanser until you can replace it. Also, make sure your face is wet before applying. Scrub can feel very abrasive on dry skin.

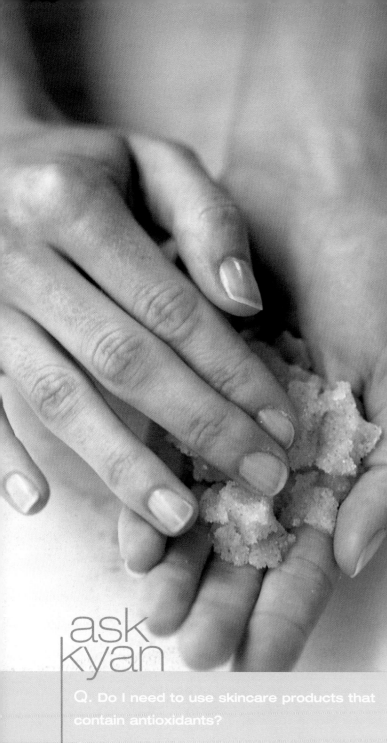

acids). You'll find them in certain moisturizers, cleansers, toners, and at-home peels. Doctors use these acids for in-office procedures, such as in chemical peels, but in stronger concentrations than are available commercially.

You can use a moisturizer, cleanser, or toner with AHAs or BHAs on a daily basis. If dry, red, or flaky patches occur when using any AHA or BHA product, you may need to stop using them or use them less frequently.

serum

This is a new product category that's pretty misunderstood. Many people think serums are moisturizers, but that's not always the case. Some do add moisture or can be used instead of moisturizer, but most are meant as a treatment to be used *under* moisturizer. Generally, serums provide an antioxidant boost, deliver other anti-aging ingredients, vitamins, or nutrients, or lighten the skin.

Do you absolutely need a serum? No, but if you want a little something extra for your skin, go ahead and give it a try.

super scrub

Mix some exfoliating scrub into your mud or clay mask for a super-cleansing facial. Gently massage onto your face, then let dry. Remove by alternately splashing your face with lukewarm water and massaging off the product.

moisturizer

Simply put, a moisturizer softens and sometimes draws moisture to the skin. It comes in cream, lotion, and gel formulas, creams being the heaviest and gels being the lightest. A

ask kyan

Q. Do I need to use skincare products that contain antioxidants?

A. If you want to prevent wrinkles, it's a great idea to use a moisturizer or serum that contains antioxidants. In case you weren't paying attention in chemistry class, antioxidants protect against free radicals, which are atoms or molecules with unpaired electrons. They literally bounce around looking to steal the necessary electrons, wreaking havoc on your skin and advancing the signs of aging. Free radicals are exacerbated by smoking, pollution, and sunlight. Antioxidants are your best defense.

moisturizer can be plain and simple, or it can be packed with anti-aging ingredients. A basic moisturizer moisturizes. That's it. It will not prevent, fade, or reduce wrinkles unless it contains anti-aging ingredients. A good ingredient to look for is hyaluronic acid, a natural substance that is an excellent moisturizing agent.

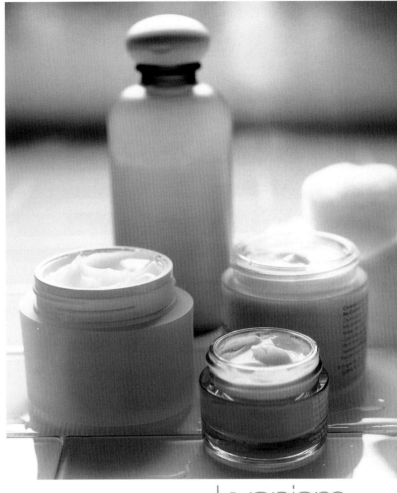

eye cream

If you're in your teens, you do not need eye cream, but once you're in your twenties, it's a great product to incorporate into your routine.

Selecting an eye cream can be confusing because there are so many different types on the market. Some do nothing but add a layer of moisture to the under-eye area. I find these rather redundant if you already use moisturizer. A better choice is a problem-specific eye cream. Choose one that addresses morning puffiness, dark circles, or fine lines, whichever is your issue.

Use your ring finger to gently dot eye cream over your moisturizer. Don't get too close to the lashline. I don't like to put eye cream on my upper eyelids, but if yours are dry or crepey, eye cream will help.

Don't go overboard with the eye cream. I find that I break out when I use too much. Also, excessive usage can lead to millia, those little whiteheads that need to be removed by a dermatologist.

pore strips

Are these the best things ever or what? I have a neurotic obsession with pore strips. There's something so addictive about investigating the junk attached to the strip once you've pulled if off your face. It's like a weird topographical map with all these tiny craters and mountains.

When using, follow the directions and let the strip dry completely. Don't use pore strips more than once a week; more frequent use could irritate your skin.

kyanism

Keep Those Crow's Feet at Bay Want to prevent wrinkles around your eyes? Eye cream's not the answer; staying out of the sun is. Wear sunscreen every day and wear sunglasses that protect the eye area every time you're outside. If reduction is your issue, not prevention, try an eye cream that promises to reduce or fade wrinkles or fine lines.

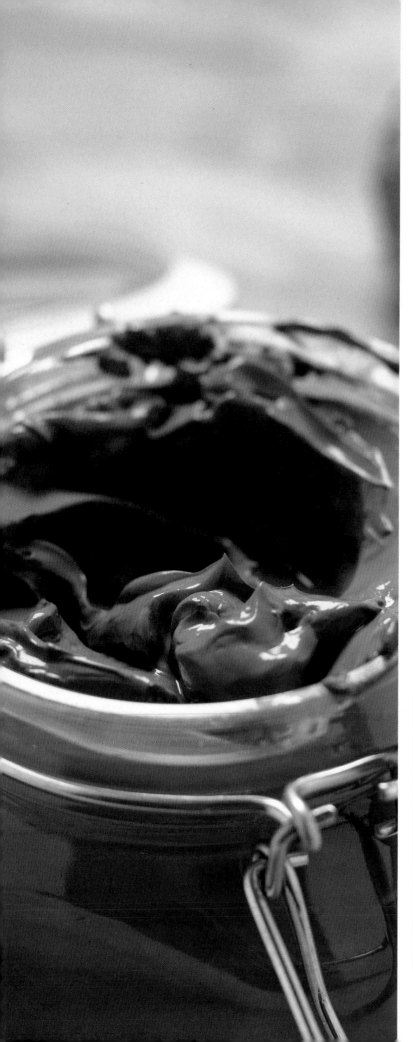

masks One of the best ways to pamper yourself and treat your skin at the same time is with a face mask. It doesn't matter whether you do it at home, or you go to a spa or a salon.

- purifying masks These draw out impurities and are great for oily or combination skin. Made of such ingredients as clay and mud, they generally dry out your skin, causing a tightening feeling as the mask dries. Wear until the mask dries completely or for as long as directed. Rinse off with lukewarm water.

- hydrating masks These add moisture and soften dry skin. Different ingredients include aloe, avocado, shea butter, and jojoba. Leave on for 15 minutes or as directed. Remove with tissues or lukewarm water.

- exfoliating masks These brighten, tighten, and smooth the skin. They often contain natural exfoliants such as pumpkin or papaya. They can be used by most skin types (people with sensitive skin types should be careful); read the label to be sure.

the spa facial

Some facials are incredibly pampering and gentle; others can be a bit rough, especially if they involve extractions, a process in which blackheads and other congested matter are manually removed from your pores. Extractions might leave you with lots of little red spots that will take a few days to heal. Don't get extractions right before a big date or event.

steam clean

It's great to steam your face and open your pores before applying a mask. Boil some water in a pot, remove from the heat, and lean over the pot. Your face should be at least 12 inches away from the water. You're looking to gently steam your skin, not cook it! The process should not be painful. Steam for 15 seconds.

For an aromatherapy boost, add a few drops of essential oil or a chamomile or peppermint teabag to the water.

d.i.y.

Several years ago, when I was on my own and living in New Orleans, I loved making skincare products from scratch. I'd throw some ingredients into a blender and whip up some face masks or scrubs. Somehow I always found willing guinea pigs to test these homemade concoctions, and their complexions did seem to benefit from them.

It's really easy to make your own face mask with ingredients like bananas, avocado, oatmeal, eggs, or yogurt. Try the product on the inside of your elbow before applying to your face, just to make sure you have no skin allergies to any ingredients. If any product ever stings or turns your skin red, wash it off immediately.

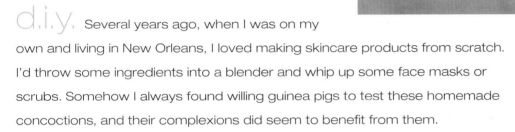

KYAN'S FAVORITE FACE MASK

Here's a great recipe for soothing dry skin.

INGREDIENTS

Half an avocado
Half a banana
¼ cup oatmeal

MASH ALL THE INGREDIENTS together in a bowl using a potato masher or a fork. Get all the bumps out. Apply to your freshly washed face. Leave on for 10 minutes, then rinse. Pat your face dry. Apply moisturizer if necessary.

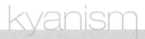

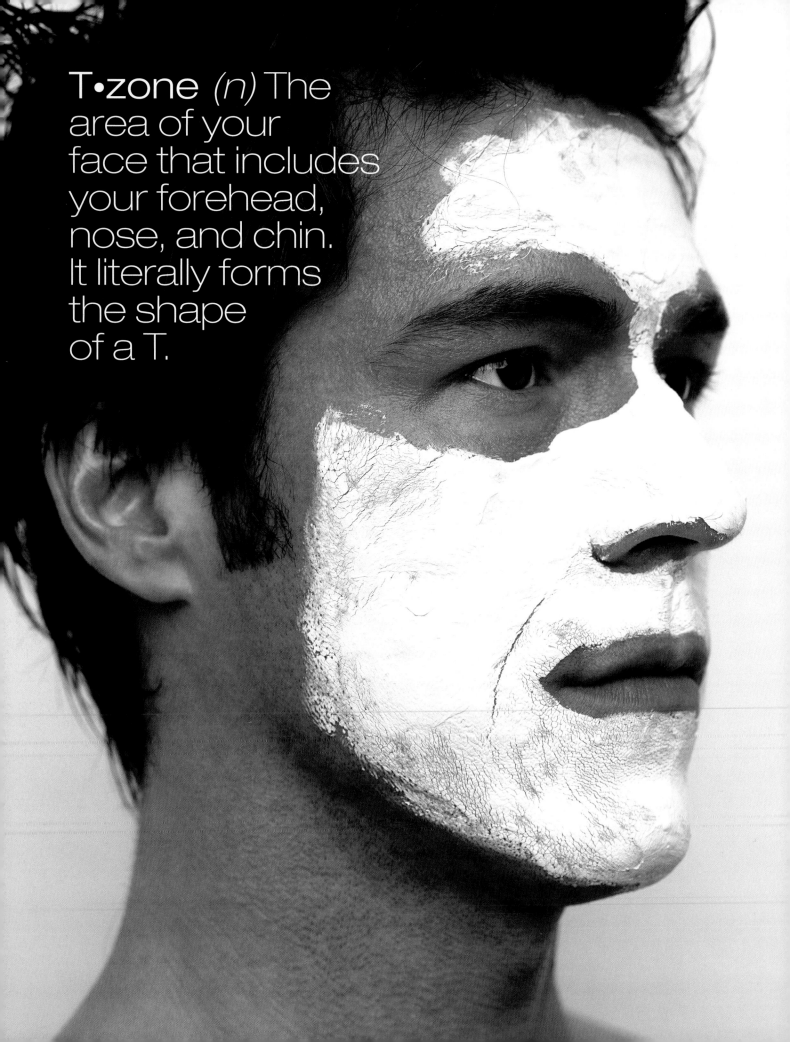

T•zone *(n)* The area of your face that includes your forehead, nose, and chin. It literally forms the shape of a T.

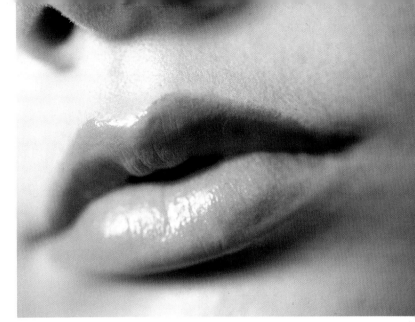

lip balms and exfoliants

Would you want to kiss someone with dry, chapped lips? I know I wouldn't. Lips are a good measure of your hydration level. If they get dry a lot, you're probably not drinking enough water. Eight ounces of water eight times day is a must.

Your lips should be soft and supple. Make sure that you always have some lip balm on hand and use it throughout the day. If you're going to be outside, make sure it has an SPF. I'm not a fan of petroleum-based balms, because the molecules are too big to be absorbed. Try natural balms, especially ones made of shea butter. Waxy balms? Toss them.

If your lips are dry and chapped, you need to exfoliate them. Some people use a toothbrush or washcloth, but I think it's better to use something more gentle. Try one of the lip exfoliation products on the market. Or better yet, make your own.

SWEET AND SIMPLE LIP SCRUB

INGREDIENTS

½ teaspoon white sugar
½ teaspoon olive oil

MIX THE INGREDIENTS in the palm of your hand, rub on your lips, then rinse off with a little water. Pat your lips dry, then apply some balm.

kyanism

Go Natural I love anything organic and environmentally friendly, and I think it's great to seek out products like this. Keep in mind, however, that just because it's natural doesn't mean it's gentle. Some of these products contain essential oils that are too strong for sensitive skin. Try to sample the product before buying, if possible.

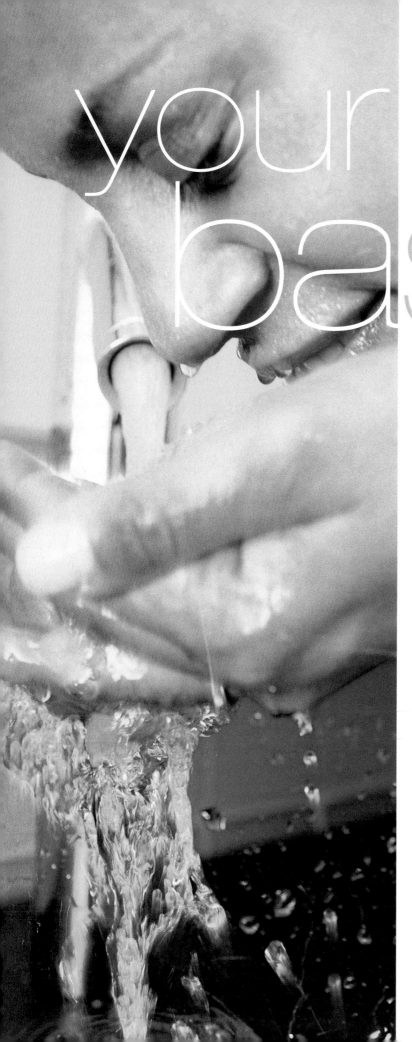

your basic routine

normal skin

a.m. Wash your face with a mild foaming cleanser or splash your face with lukewarm water.

Moisturize with a lightweight lotion. You might want a heavier lotion or cream in the colder months or if you live in a dry climate. Apply eye cream if necessary.

Apply sunscreen 15 to 30 minutes before leaving the house.

p.m. Wash your face with a mild foaming cleanser. If this isn't enough to take off your makeup, use makeup remover cloths or liquid remover and cotton balls first, followed by cleanser.

Use a treatment-packed moisturizer based on your skincare needs (wrinkle prevention, acne prevention, radiance boosting, etc.). Follow with eye cream if necessary.

Exfoliate with a face scrub every week.

dry skin

a.m. Splash your face with lukewarm water.

Moisturize with a lotion or cream, depending on your preference and level of dryness. Follow with eye cream if necessary.

Apply sunscreen 15 to 30 minutes before leaving the house.

p.m. Wash your face with a creamy cleanser that does not foam. If this isn't enough to take off your makeup, try makeup remover cloths or liquid remover and cotton balls first, followed by the cleanser.

Use a treatment-packed moisturizer based on your skincare needs (wrinkle prevention, acne prevention, radiance boosting, etc.). Follow with eye cream.

Exfoliate with a face scrub every week or two.

oily skin

a.m. Wash your face with a foaming gel cleanser.

Apply toner using a cotton ball or pad. (You can skip this step and use only in the evening if you like.)

Moisturize with an oil-free lotion, if necessary. Use eye cream if you like.

Apply an oil-free sunscreen 15 to 30 minutes before leaving the house.

p.m. Wash your face with a foaming gel cleanser.

Apply toner using a cotton ball or pad.

Moisturize with a light treatment-packed lotion, if necessary. Something with AHAs or BHAs is a good choice to prevent acne and promote cell turnover. Use eye cream if you like.

Exfoliate with a scrub two to three times a week.

Use a clay or mud mask once a week.

combination skin

a.m. Wash your face with a foaming gel cleanser. If your skin feels tight, switch to a nonfoaming creamy cleanser or a foaming cleanser formulated for dry skin.

Moisturize with a lightweight lotion. If that doesn't do the trick, switch to something heavier, or just spot treat the dry areas with something richer. Apply eye cream if necessary.

Apply sunscreen 15 to 30 minutes before leaving the house.

p.m. Wash your face with the cleanser of your choice.

Moisturize with a lightweight, treatment-packed lotion. If that doesn't produce the results you want, switch to something heavier, or spot treat the dry areas with something richer. Apply eye cream if necessary.

Exfoliate with a face scrub once a week.

Use a clay or mud mask on your nose or T-zone once a week.

sensitive skin

It seems as if more and more people have sensitive skin these days. If you fall into this category, use products formulated for sensitive skin or ones that are free of fragrance, color, AHAs, and BHAs.

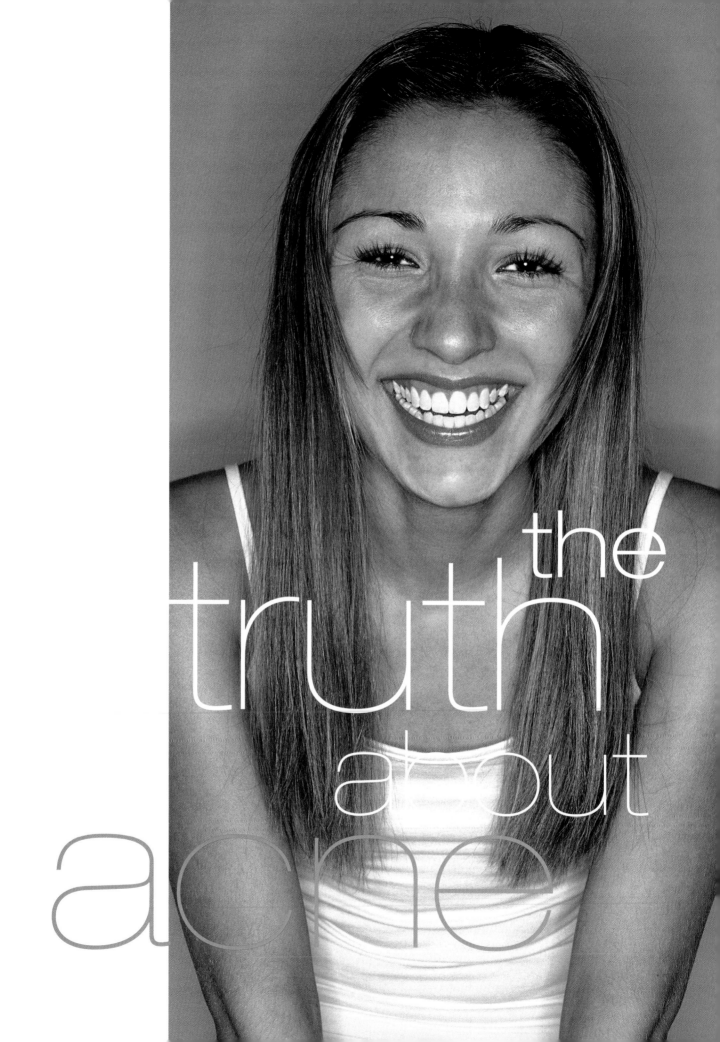

the
truth
about
acne

Do you get the occasional pimple? Do you break out once a month, right before your period? If this describes your condition, you have mild acne and might be able to treat yourself with over-the-counter products. But if you have painful, intense blemishes or are embarrassed by your skin, then you need to see a professional. Don't suffer—seek help.

Acne is a disease. Nobody gets it because he or she is bad or lazy or has a rotten diet—its causes are primarily factors you can't control. Granted, you're not doing yourself any favors if you exist solely on candy, fast food, and soda. These may exacerbate your condition, but they're not solely the reason for your bad skin. Plenty of people have bad habits and never get pimples.

If you're one of the lucky few with amazing skin, count your blessings and don't ever judge or make fun of someone because of his or her skin. If you're not so lucky, don't despair. I know severe acne can be terrible emotionally and socially, but you need to be strong, take control of the situation, and find a solution. There are now more effective treatments for acne than ever before.

In this section, I'll cover the products and procedures you can use to get better skin, but if you're really unhappy about a skin-related issue, you should see a dermatologist. These doctors specialize in skin (and hair and nails as well) and can recommend treatments or medications that will improve your skin's condition. Health insurance often covers visits to the dermatologist, so check

accutane should always be taken under the supervision of a doctor. Don't buy it online or use someone else's prescription!

kyanism

Too Hot! Always wash your face with lukewarm water. Hot water is too extreme for facial skin.

the doctor is in

I've asked my friend and dermatologist, Dr. Brad Katchen, for his help in understanding acne and finding the best treatments. Dr. Katchen's clients include movie stars who have to see their faces magnified a thousand times on the big screen (terrifying, no?), so you're in good hands with him.

Kyan: So what causes acne?

Dr. Katchen: It's generally hormones, stress, and genetics. There's a huge genetic predisposition to acne. Technically, it all starts at the intersection where the hair follicle and oil gland come together. There's an issue with the turnover of the cells that line the follicle. The follicle gets clogged with those cells and that's how you get an inflammatory acne lesion, also know as a pimple.

Kyan: Why do some pimples become whiteheads?

Dr. Katchen: Because inflammatory cells have flocked to the area to fight the acne. The pus that results consists of these cells.

Kyan: What is a blackhead?

Dr. Katchen: It's a clogged pore, which is another type of acne lesion. Most people think blackheads have something to do with dirt or not cleansing their faces well enough, but the color comes from the pigment, also known as melanin, that's produced both in the hair follicles and the cells that line the follicle.

Kyan: Is benzoyl peroxide a good quick fix?

Dr. Katchen: It's a good spot treatment. Use a small amount, because too much can

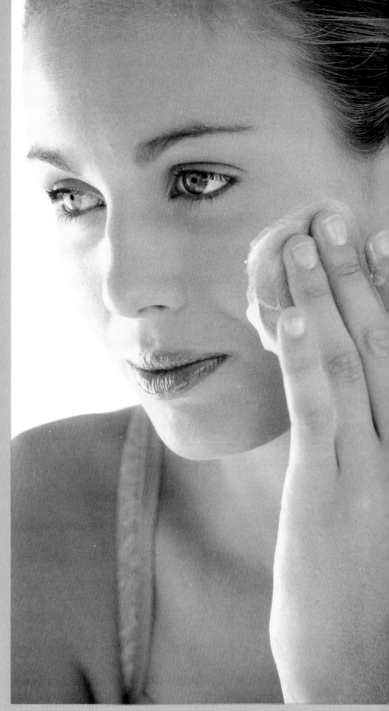

dry out your skin and even irritate sensitive skin. Also, keep in mind that it can bleach clothing, towels, and sheets if it comes in contact with them.

Kyan: What about salicylic acid? A lot of acne products contain that today.

Dr. Katchen: It's not as good a drying agent as benzoyl peroxide, but it can function as an anti-inflammatory. It's best as an exfoliating ingredient for acne-prone skin.

your policy. If your dermatologist recommends a prescription product that is too pricey, ask for a cheaper over-the-counter option instead.

If a doctor's visit is impossible for whatever reason, you need to educate yourself. Go online, borrow some skincare books from the library, or visit an alternative bookstore to investigate natural remedies. Anything you do to educate yourself will give you control over the situation and take away some of the emotional angst associated with acne and other skin disorders.

Initially, your doctor will probably recommend benzoyl peroxide. Products with this medicated ingredient help to destroy acne-causing bacteria and can be used to dry up existing acne or prevent future flare-ups. It is available in different strengths, either as an over-the-counter product or as a prescription.

other acne treatments

retin-a This drug, available by prescription only, speeds up the natural exfoliation process and helps prevent clogged pores. This is best for acne prevention. Using too much Retin-A can lead to redness and severely dry skin. Carefully follow your doctor's instructions for usage.

Retin-A is expensive and requires a prescription, but there are other over-the-counter products, like retinols, that can also be used instead (although they're not necessarily as effective). You also can select something with AHAs or BHAs to help with cell turnover.

accutane Also available by prescription only, this drug clears up serious acne and can prevent future breakouts. In fact, doctors generally believe that Accutane is the only medicine that has the potential to cure acne. It works wonders for people with chronic cystic acne, and it will help prevent the scarring associated with that type of acne. Because of the potential side effects, however, you need to be well monitored by your doctor while on the drug throughout the course of treatment.

The results of Accutane are often amazing, but if you're taking it you must be careful about how much alcohol you drink. In addition, you must be very conscientious about birth control if you're sexually active because Accutane can cause birth defects. You cannot get laser treatments while on Accutane. The combination can result in scarring. If you're getting waxed, tell your esthetician you're taking the drug. He or she needs to be cautious because your skin will be more sensitive.

kyanism

Scrub Straight Talk
If you have active acne, you shouldn't use a face scrub. It will only aggravate your condition. Instead, use an exfoliating product every day or a weekly mask containing AHAs or BHAs.

the doctor is in

Kyan: Which ingredient is better for peels, AHAs or BHAs?

Dr. Katchen: I prefer BHAs, in particular salicylic acid. BHAs penetrate the hair follicle and you get a better exfoliation. Plus, you get a more uniform reaction. With glycolic acid peels, you sometimes get hot spots, which are irritated patches on the face.

Kyan: What do you think of at-home chemical peels?

Dr. Katchen: I'm not a fan. If the chemicals get into your eyes, you could be in big trouble. If you leave certain peels on your face for too long, you could cause inflammation. Lastly, some people with dry, flaky, inflamed skin think they should peel it and the inflammation will be gone, but that's totally wrong. They just make the problem worse.

laser precautions

- Don't have a treatment after you've been in the sun. It can cause permanent discoloration of your skin.
- Protect your eyes as directed. These treatments can seriously impair your vision.

ask kyan

Q. Why can't I pick at my pimples? Everyone else does, right? Surely you have.

A. Of course I have, but now that I know better, I don't. It's a bad habit to get into. It will make your pimple look worse and can cause infection and scarring. If you find yourself picking at your skin obsessively, you could have a problem. If that's the case, talk to your doctor.

In rare circumstances, Accutane can also cause serious emotional side effects, so have a frank discussion with your doctor before starting treatment. Make sure to do your own research and come to your doctor's appointment armed with questions before agreeing to a prescription.

chemical peels These are a great way to clean out clogged pores and prevent pimples. Your dermatologist can give you a peel in his or her office or you can do an at-home peel. However, the at-home variety is not as concentrated and powerful as those administered in a doctor's office.

lasers Certain lasers can target and kill the bacteria that cause pimples and lessen the occurrence of future acne. Intense pulsed light, or IPL, is a similar treatment that gets lumped into the laser category. Both tend to be very expensive.

Lasers also are used today to stimulate collagen production, reduce redness, fade brown spots, acne scars, and broken capillaries, reduce hair growth, and remove tattoos (which we'll discuss at the end of this chapter). These treatments can be very expensive. Some require zero downtime, others require a longer recovery. Certain laser treatments do not work on dark skin tones.

Doctors can do laser treatments, and there are lots of skincare centers that do the treatments at a lower cost. If you get a laser treatment at one of these centers, make sure the person using the laser is certified and supervised.

acne scars Picking at your pimples can cause scarring, but often scars develop on their own as the result of severe acne. If your scars are serious, you'll need to see a dermatologist.

Treatments for scarring include chemical peels, dermabrasion, micro-dermabrasion, laser resurfacing, and collagen injections. The costs and recovery time vary for all these options, so talk to your doctor about what's best for your condition, your schedule, and your pocketbook.

emergency zit zapping

Let's say you've got a major event coming up—the prom, a job interview, your wedding, whatever—and right before the big day, it happens. A giant red pimple. Before you plunge into despair, call your dermatologist. He or she can inject it with cortisone and it should disappear within 24 hours.

back to basics

If you've got acne, remember that healthy living will make a difference. Making positive changes in your diet, drinking plenty of water, and getting enough sleep will help.

stressed-out skin

Everybody's stressed. Sadly, it seems to be the normal state of affairs these days. If you've got a mysterious skin condition or an unusually bad case of acne, stress could be to blame. It's proven that stress exacerbates or even causes skin problems like acne, psoriasis, and dandruff. The lesson: Get your stress under control. Your skin will thank you.

zapping zits

Lets review:

- To spot treat pimples, try a benzoyl peroxide product.
- To prevent future acne, treat breakout-prone areas with salicylic acid products.
- For serious cystic acne, see your dermatologist.

ask kyan

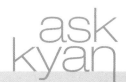

Q. When I'm stressed, I break out around my mouth. How can I prevent this?

A. Try meditation and relaxation techniques (see pages 200–203). Stress plays a huge role in breakouts, so if you can keep your stress to a minimum, drink lots of water, and keep your hands off your face, you'll have a better time at keeping your skin under control.

P.S. Pimples around your mouth and chin are often caused by pressing your phone against your face. Make sure to clean your phone regularly and hold it near your face, but don't let it touch it. Believe it or not, your phone is a powerful transmittor of bacteria, dirt, and oil.

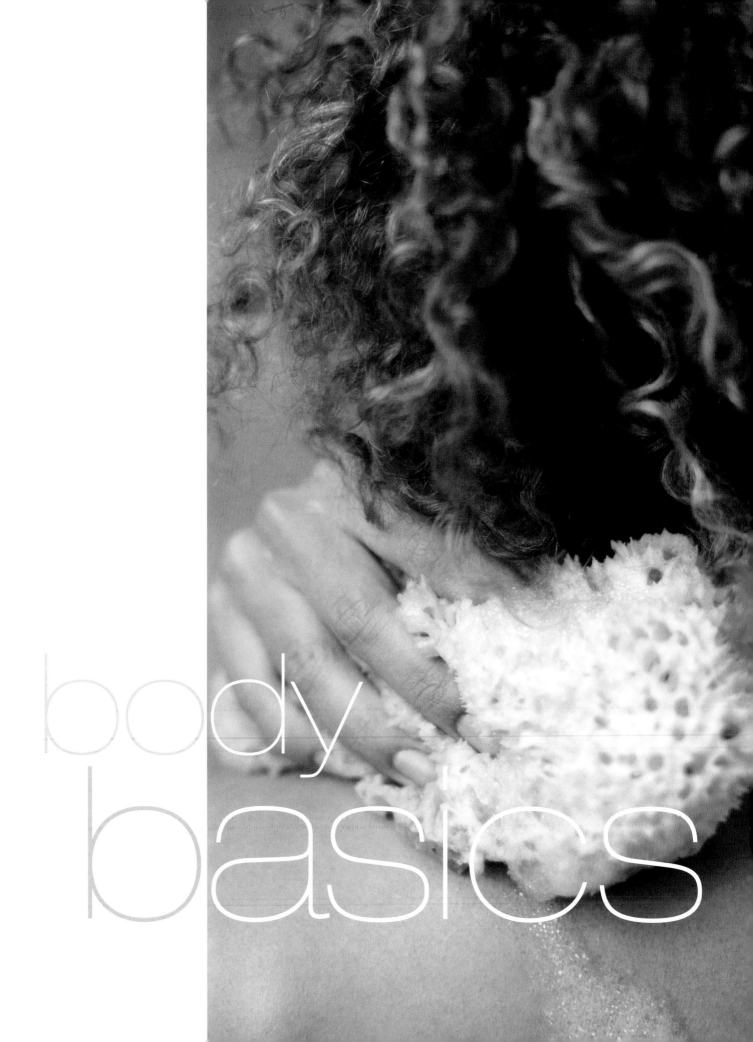

body
basics

Everybody knows that your skin doesn't begin with your forehead and end at your chin, yet that's the area everyone concentrates on the most. You need to take care of your skin from head to toe.

- Consider your ears, neck, shoulders, and chest an extension of your facial skin and treat accordingly.
- Your chest and shoulders are very prone to sunburn, so protect them with sunscreen when outdoors.
- Your hands give away your age faster than your face. Use a hand cream with SPF throughout the day.
- Apply body lotion after every bath or shower.
- Exfoliate your knees, elbows, and feet regularly. Follow with a rich moisturizer.
- Exfoliate your body and boost your circulation by stroking your skin with a dry brush. (Buy a soft body brush at a drugstore or health food store.) You can do this every morning before you get in the shower. Brush toward your heart, not away from it.
- If bacne (acne on your back) is a problem, cleanse with a specially formulated body wash. Since the back is hard to reach, try to find a salicylic body spray to treat the area.

my desert island skincare

If I were going to be stranded, I'd want a cleanser, a moisturizer with SPF, and a lip balm with SPF.

sunscreen

Growing up in Florida, I was tan all the time. My family, like most back then, wasn't educated about sun damage, so we ran around without a trace of sunscreen on our bodies. The only people who did were the hot lifeguards with the thick, white stripes of zinc oxide protecting their noses. Today, my freckled shoulders are the only evidence of my beach bum days, thank God. It's a proven fact that excessive sun exposure ages the skin prematurely and is the leading cause of skin cancer, the most common form of cancer in the United States.

Now I never leave the house without sunscreen. Whether you use a moisturizer with SPF or a separate sunscreen, some level of protection is a must. The earlier you start minimizing your exposure and protecting yourself, the better. Believe it or not, the majority of your sun exposure—and damage—has occurred by the

ask kyan

Q. Do I need to wear sunscreen in the winter?

A. Absolutely. Just because you're not lying out in your favorite bikini doesn't mean that you're not exposed to ultraviolet rays. A walk to the grocery store, a drive to a friend's house, the short trip to the subway, anytime you're outside, you're getting exposed. Today, when tons of moisturizers contain sunscreen, there is no excuse for going unprotected.

time you turn eighteen. That said, it's never too late to start being smart about the sun.

Wearing a cool hat is a smart and stylish way of protecting your face from the sun. (But don't think that wearing one means that you don't need to wear sunscreen, too!) Wide-brimmed, floppy straw hats can be really cute. But if you wear a woven straw hat, make sure that it's dense enough so that it actually blocks your face from the sun. If it's made of a loose weave, the sun can shine straight through its holes, even if they seem really tiny. Make sure your hat casts complete shade over your face.

how to choose the right sunscreen

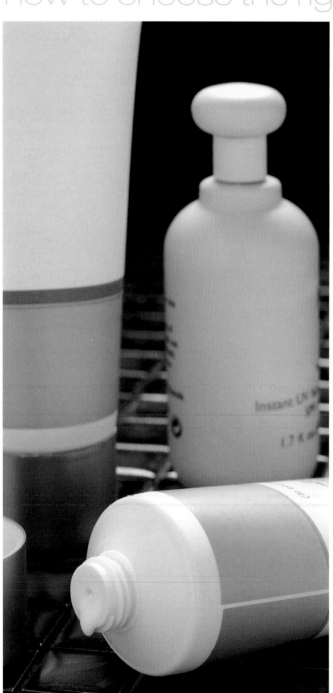

Always use SPF 15 or higher. You want a broad-spectrum formula, meaning that it protects against both UVA and UVB rays.

chemical block These sunscreens have ingredients that absorb ultraviolet radiation and, as a result, prevent your skin from soaking up the rays. The best ingredient to look for is called Parsol 1789.

physical block These sunscreens have ingredients that deflect the sun's rays. Look for things like zinc oxide and titanium dioxide. In the past, these sunscreens tended to be heavy and chalky. Today, thanks to ingredients like micronized zinc oxide, they're much lighter, less sticky, and easier to wear.

Whether you prefer a chemical or physical block is up to you. If you find that chemical sunscreen aggravates your skin, you could be allergic to it. Try a physical block instead.

Apply your sunscreen 15 to 30 minutes before going outside. If you're spending the day outside, reapply liberally every hour or two.

Sunscreen expires. Once a year, throw away all your sunscreen! (P.S. If you have any sunscreen left over from the previous summer, chances are you didn't use enough.)

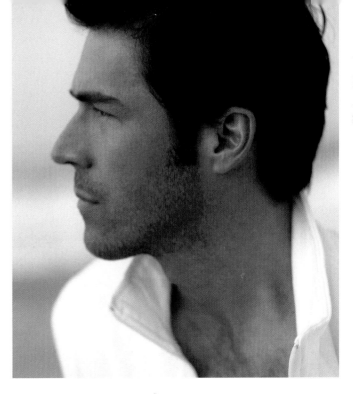

fake it, don't bake it

You already know how damaging the sun can be on your skin, and that you need to protect yourself with sunscreen. But what if you happen to look and feel better with a tan? The solution is self-tanner. Today's formulas are so easy to use and natural looking, there's no excuse for baking on the beach.

self-tanner tips

- If you're a beginner, use a formula for light skin tones. (Some brands have light, medium, and dark formulas; some are "one color fits all.") Be sure to apply the least amount as possible, and you'll learn how much to use as you familiarize yourself with the effects it has on your skin.
- Exfoliate before you begin.
- Do not moisturize before applying, with the exception of your elbows, knees, heels, and ankles. The skin in these areas tends to be dry, so self-tanner likes to stick there. Moisturizing these spots in advance will result in a smooth and even application. You'll notice that these areas look darker on amateur self-tanners.
- Use disposable plastic gloves to apply self-tanner.
- Avoid getting the product on your fingernails and toenails.
- Be careful around your hairline and eyebrows. Make sure you apply to skin where hairlines begin. Amateur self-tanners often don't get as close to the hairline as necessary.
- Don't forget your ears.
- Don't be heavy-handed. You can always apply a second coat later.
- When finished, remove your gloves and apply self-tanner to the backs of your hands. Gently rub the backs and the sides of your hands together. Skip your palms. No one has tanned palms.
- Don't have gloves? Wash your hands a few times throughout the process. When you're finished applying, wash your hands with body scrub.
- Be as naked as possible when self-tanning.
- Let the product dry and set as directions indicate before getting dressed. Don't wear white right away if you can avoid it.
- When you shower, soap up your body with your hands. A washcloth will remove your self-tanner prematurely. Exfoliant will remove even more.
- Moisturize your body every day to prolong your tan.
- Reapply a bit of self-tanner to the backs of your hands as needed. Because you wash your hands frequently (or at least I hope you do), the color wears away faster than on the rest of your body. You want to have even coloring at all times.

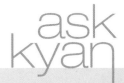

ask kyan

Q. Is olive oil really an effective moisturizer?

A. It is, but I'd recommend using it on your elbows, knees, and other dry spots—not on your face.

ouch!

Let's say you somehow managed to get a sunburn. Maybe you didn't realize you'd be outside, or you didn't wear enough sunscreen. It happens. When you get home, apply an over-the-counter hydracortisone cream (it's an anti-inflammatory). Following that, you might want to apply a cool compress. For the rest of the week, make sure you moisturize with something gentle and soothing. Anything highly fragranced or really active might irritate your skin further. Be sure to wash your skin as infrequently as possible and use mild soap. Washing too often will dry out your skin and result in excessive peeling.

Do not exfoliate until the redness has disappeared and the peeling has stopped. If you have blisters, let them heal. Don't pick at them. Today, when information about the damaging effects of sun exposure is so readily available, sunburns can be really embarrassing. Proper care will allow for faster healing.

ask kyan

Q. What can I put on my skin to prevent scarring?
A. The effects of scarring can be reduced with vitamin E. (I recommend this not for use on your face, but elsewhere on your body.) Once your wound is healed, apply concentrated, liquid vitamin E. There are also over-the-counter scar guards and ointments.

a fine mist

Can't get the hang of self-tanning yourself? Here are some other options.

spray tan You stand in a booth wearing as little as possible while a machine mists you from head to toe. I did this and the results were great, except that my feet got coated with too much product because all the mist falls to the floor. Next time, I'd wear a pair of socks I could throw away and self-tan my feet afterward.

airbrush tan An esthetician sprays you from head to toe using a hand-held airbrush machine. If the esthetician is really experienced, he or she can use the tanning solution to give you the illusion of more emphasized cheekbones and sculpted abs. This is the more expensive option because of the labor and time involved.

bed time Tanning beds are not a good idea. Most people don't wear protection when using them, and you have no idea what kind of bulbs are used. They also seem to result in tans with an orange tint that are obviously artificial. Try spray or airbrush tanning instead.

skin cancer screening

If you're between the ages of 20 and 39, the American Cancer Society recommends that you get a skin checkup every three years to make sure you don't have any suspicious moles, freckles, or blemishes. If you're 40 or over, you should visit your dermatologist for a screening every year. Regardless of your age, do a thorough check of your skin once a month. Call your doctor if anything has changed in color or shape, is bleeding, or is itchy.

quick fixes?

Want plumper lips? Fuller cheeks? Fewer wrinkles? Smoother skin? These can be achieved through procedures that fall under the heading of cosmetic dermatology—cosmetic because they're medically unnecessary, but they help improve one's appearance. They're often called quick fixes, because in comparison to plastic surgery, they take a fraction of the time. However, I think that term plays down the effort, pain, and high prices involved.

Here are a few of these services you can get from a dermatologist or plastic surgeon.

botox

Everybody's talking about Botox these days. Basically, it's a neurotoxin injected into the face or neck to soften the appearance of wrinkles. It works by reducing the muscle contractions that cause your skin to crease, essentially freezing parts of your face so you can't make certain expressions, like furrowing your brow or wrinkling your forehead. The Food & Drug Administration has approved Botox for use between the eyebrows, but doctors are using it in various ways—on the forehead, to raise the tip of the nose, to reduce wrinkles on the neck, even to cure migraines.

Pain-wary patients can have the injection site numbed first. Minor bruising may result. Botox takes a few days to kick in and lasts about three months.

collagen

Think movie stars are born with full, plump lips? Not all of them. Some get their pouts loaded up with collagen. While this substance is naturally occurring in human skin, the kind that doctors use comes from cows, believe it or not. (They refer to it as bovine collagen.) Collagen can also be used to fill in acne scars, wrinkles, and other depressions in the face.

restylane

This is becoming more popular than collagen for adding volume to the face, plumping lips, and filling wrinkles. It's derived from hyaluronic acid, a naturally occuring substance in the body. Bruising, swelling, itching, and/or tenderness can occur as a result of a Restylane injection.

Fish Lips

We've all seen people with too much collagen in their lips. It's not a pretty sight. If collagen is what you want, tell your doctor you'd like a subtle enhancement, not a mouth you can see from a block away.

kyanism

Mixed Feelings
Botox, although FDA approved, is a toxin. I don't know how much I like the idea of introducing a toxin into my system. I'd recommend researching Botox extensively and discussing it with a few trusted professionals before deciding to do it. Although we know the visual effects last only several months, there may be long-term effects that haven't been discovered yet.

piercing dos and don'ts

. . . **don't** let your friends pierce any part of you. Piercings are very prone to infection, and an amateur job is a great way to guarantee trouble.

. . . **do** find a professional to do the job, and make sure the workspace is clean and the tools sterilized. If not, find another pro.

tattoo don'ts

You know I don't like to tell anyone how to live his or her life, but . . .

. . . **don't** ever let a friend give you a tattoo. Not only will it not look as good as a trained artist's, it could result in permanent scarring or even life-threatening disease.

. . . **don't** ever get a tattoo on your face, hands, or neck. You might not realize it now, but you're seriously limiting your future employment opportunities. People often find visible tattoos threatening or off-putting.

. . . **don't** have the name of a significant other tattooed on you. There are lots of ways to say "I love you," and a tattoo shouldn't be one of them. The name of your mother, father, children, or beloved pet are fine, but other people tend to come in and out of our lives. We think some relationships will last forever, yet they don't always. Sorry to be so harsh.

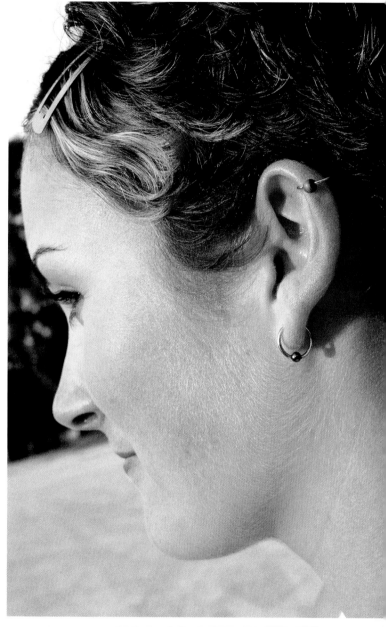

tattoo you

When I was 18, I got a small spider tattooed on my chest. I had seen a picture of some guy in a magazine with the tattoo and thought it was the coolest thing ever, so I had to have one. I didn't go to a tattoo parlor; rather, this guy named Scott did it in his living room. If I had to do it over again, I wouldn't, but I'm not about to remove it. I like my little jailhouse tattoo. It brings back a lot of memories, and besides, my mistakes are part of who I am. I don't want to go back and erase them.

That said, if you want a tattoo, here are a few things to keep in mind:

• Get tattoo artist recommendations from people whose tattoos you like.

• Make sure the artist's workspace is clean and the tools are sterilized. If you're uncomfortable with the setup, leave.

• Put a lot of thought into the design you want. Make sure it's meaningful, expressive, and personal. Is it something you'll be proud of in ten years? Is it something that really represents who you are?

caring for your tattoo

Before you leave the tattoo parlor, get specific instructions from the tattoo artist on how to care for your new design. Some artists recommend using moisturizer to help it heal, some recommend a strict regimen of antibacterial ointment. Don't pick at your tattoo while it's healing, and stay out of the sun. A good healing process can enhance the appearance and add to the life expectancy of your tattoo.

Once your tattoo has healed, moisturize the area regularly and protect it with sunscreen every time you're in the sun. Colors fade with time, and the sun will accelerate the fading process. Even with the proper maintenance, you might need a touch-up on your tattoo in a decade or so.

tattoo removal

Sick of your tattoo and want it gone? Laser is the most effective option, but it's expensive, painful, and time-consuming. (It's more expensive than the tattoo itself!) You'll need to visit the doctor at least ten to fifteen times over the course of treatment.

piercing smarts

Piercings are a great way to accessorize and assert your personality. I prefer something subtle—double-pierced ears, a small, jeweled nose piercing, a belly button ring, you get the picture. Fierce or elaborate piercings can be very intimidating, so it's important to consider what message you're sending. You might think nothing of an eyebrow ring or a pierced tongue, but others do. (Especially potential employers.) Unless you're an aspiring rock star, think twice about anything really obvious or aggressive.

caring for your piercing

Ask your piercing pro what he or she recommends. Some will tell you to apply a warm, mild mixture of water and sea salt once a day to speed the healing process. Most recommend against using hydrogen peroxide or alcohol. The saltwater mix and antibacterial soap are better solutions.

You'll have to clean your piercing a few times a day, so make sure you can commit to that before you decide to do it. Also, your hands need to be clean before you touch your piercings, so frequent hand washing is a must. If you're lazy about stuff like that—and I hope you're not—you might want to reconsider.

wake
up
your
make-
up

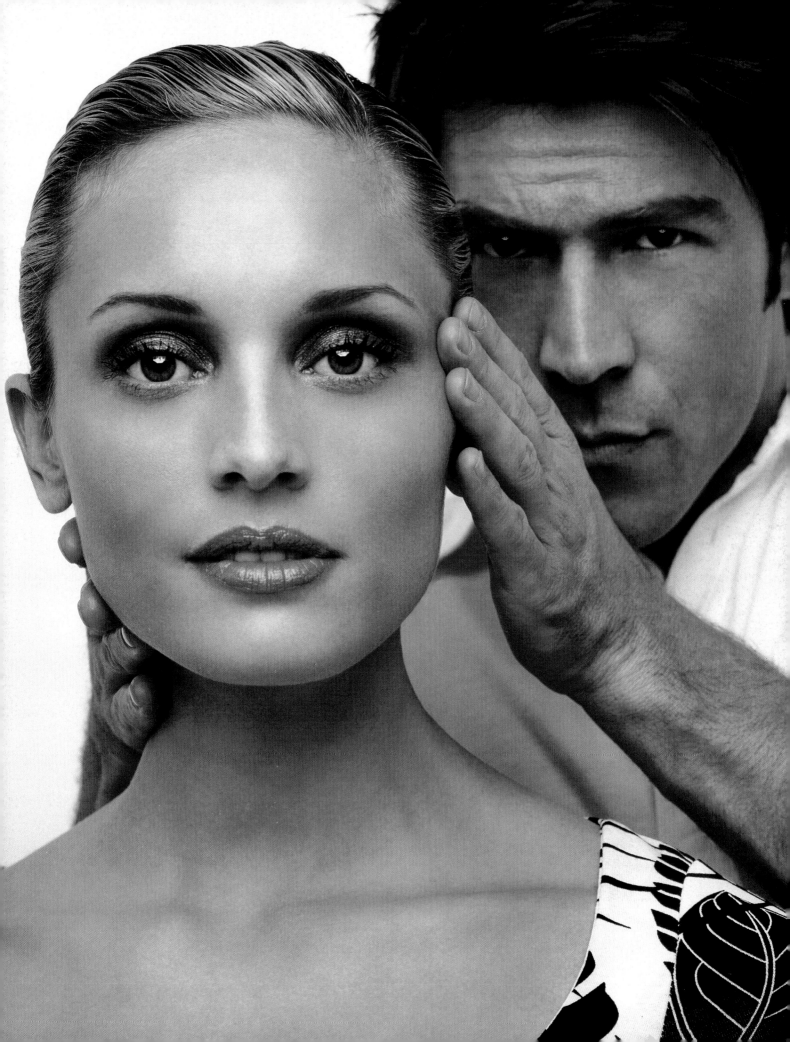

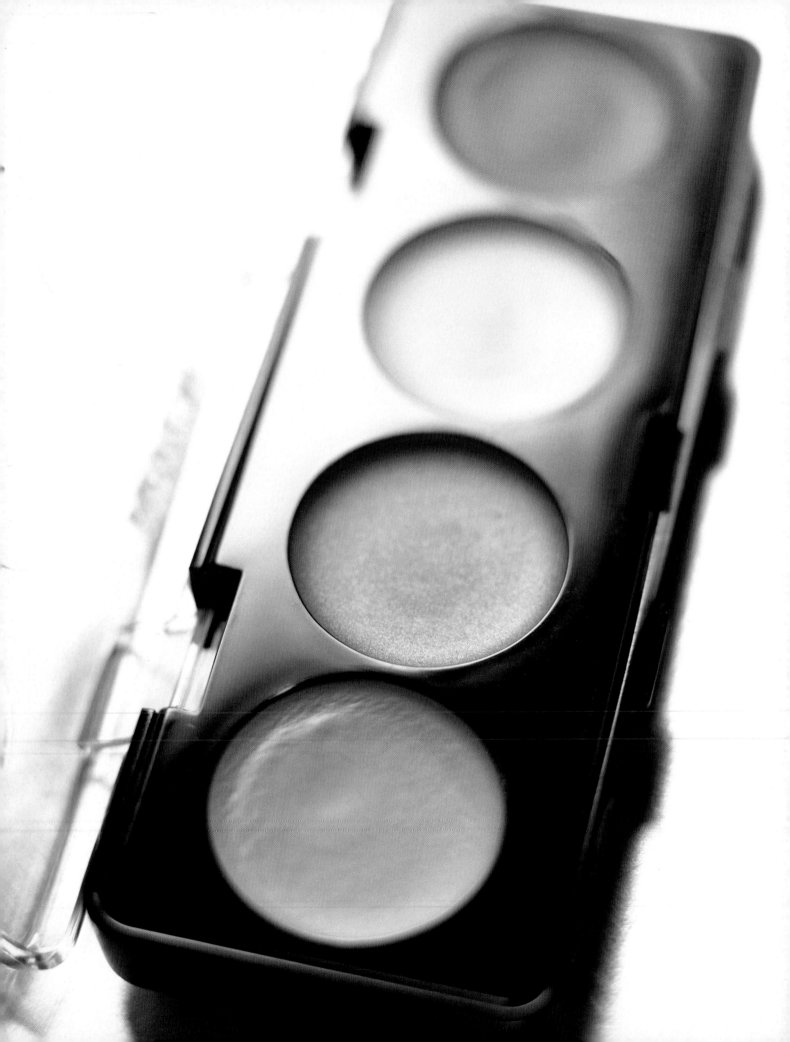

I'm going to be honest for a second here. I think that wearing makeup is a pain in the neck, but I'm saying that as a guy who has to wear it for work. The amount of light required for the TV cameras is brutal, so you need some kind of product to even out your skin tone and hide how tired you are. Off-duty, my face is makeup-free. You won't find me slapping on a little concealer before I leave the house for a soy latte. I'm tempted, but I just can't become that *guy who wears makeup.* In some ways, I feel that I'm being a little hypocritical. After all, I'm all about guys embracing themselves, having a beauty routine, using products, and all that stuff, but I can't go there. Self-tanner, exfoliants, moisturizer? Bring it on. Makeup? Sorry.

For women, however, makeup is an entirely different thing. At an early age, watching my mother do her face, I learned that makeup has the power to transform. She always put on her lipstick last, gave herself one final look in the mirror, and became a force with which to be reckoned. She became fully present and empowered. Makeup was her war paint. When you stop to think about it, women are lucky they can wear makeup. It's something that communicates your uniqueness and creativity and it's something you can have fun with, but it's also a tool for dealing with the little problems that are thrown your way. If you have a pimple, pale or blotchy skin, or a sleepless night, you can just take care of it. Getting the most out of your makeup, however, requires a certain amount of skill, knowledge, and practice.

Your look can change virtually every day, and it should. Your makeup is temporal, meaning it changes according to your mood, your outfit, the seasons—it's driven by the message that you want to send. Use it as your weapon; use it to express yourself; use it to your advantage. Mastering all the little makeup tricks that follow will allow you to become beautified. If you're unhappy with your hair one morning, pull it back and focus on making the most of your makeup instead. This is the beauty of makeup: You can design your own focal point with it, and you have absolute control over it at any given moment. If you're uneasy about going on a date or starting a new job, make sure that you're pleased with your makeup. It will put you one step closer to presenting a confident, radiant you.

In this chapter, you'll find good, solid advice and lots of extras to help you put your best face forward.

kyan's makeup shakeup checklist

assert your individuality. There's no better way to tell the world who you are than with your makeup. It's cheaper than new clothes and way less permanent and painful than tattoos or piercings.

don't hide under your makeup. Makeup should enhance your features, not re-create them. There's nothing wrong with wearing a lot of product, unless it's obvious to someone else that you're wearing a lot of product.

don't base your beauty or your self-worth on your makeup. You shouldn't be afraid to leave the house barefaced. Sure, makeup helps you feel pulled together and polished, but face it—it's not the product that makes you beautiful.

experiment! Play around with different products and brands to find what works for you. Round up your makeup, shut your bathroom or bedroom door for 10 minutes, and try out a new look or color combination.

practice makes perfect. Remember those three words. Some people are naturally better at applying makeup than others, but like anything in life, you'll never improve if you don't make an effort.

master class I think every woman should splurge on a professional makeup lesson at some point in her life. If you're new to wearing makeup, you'll get application tips and product advice, plus you'll learn what works for you. If you already wear makeup, consider it a refresher course. Ask the makeup artist to address any specific issues you have, teach you advanced tricks, like highlighting and contouring, or help you create some evening looks. No matter how much you already know, you're certain to pick up a few things.

Wondering how to find a makeup artist? Look in the phone book and call. Inquire if he or she has a portfolio of work you can view online or in person. You also can ask the salespeople at your favorite beauty counter for a recommendation. Often, the salespeople are trained as makeup artists and they'll offer to do your makeup for free. Some of them are very talented pros, while others are very

animal lover alternatives

Most makeup brushes are made from animal hair (the label might read "all-natural hair"). If you're anti-fur, look for brushes made of synthetic hair. You can find these online or at health food stores. They are just as effective as animal-hair brushes.

talented salespeople who know makeup application techniques. Before you say yes, check out the makeup they're wearing. Think they will understand you and your lifestyle? Then go for it. But remember, their job is to sell products. Most of them will take care of you in the hopes that you like the makeup and will become a customer. They might even encourage you to buy what they used. If you can't resist a sales pitch, watch out.

take stock
Before buying new makeup, take inventory of your current collection. If you've got an item you haven't worn in more than a year, toss it. Chances are you'll never wear it. Use your current collection to assess the kind of makeup wearer you are. If you've been holding on to a bottle of foundation for months and only used it once, accept that foundation isn't a necessary part of your makeup regimen and get rid of it. Cut through the clutter and focus on the products you really like and need. Once you are finished reading this chapter, you'll understand what your essentials are.

shop smart
There are so many great resources today for makeup—beauty boutiques, the Internet, catalogs, drugstores, department stores, health food stores—but where you shop really depends on your budget. I prefer places where you can test the products and ask for samples, although prices tend to be higher in stores like that.

If you shop in drugstores, where you can't sample anything, ask about the cosmetics return policy. Today, many chain drugstores will let you return makeup if the formula or the color isn't right.

tool time
I never gave much thought to makeup brushes until the makeup artist who does my face every workday lost hers. She bought an inexpensive replacement set to use until she had time to shop for some good ones, and I could really tell the difference. Not only do quality brushes feel terrific against your face, they ensure a smooth, even application of makeup.

Good brushes are expensive, but you should buy the best ones you can afford. Well-made brushes will last for years if you take good care of them. Can't afford an entire set? Buy the one or two you'll use most frequently, like a blush brush or a basic eye shadow brush.

kyanism

Dirty Girl Don't let dirty brushes touch your skin! If you use your brushes every day, gently wash them once a week in mild shampoo and warm water and let them air-dry. And please make sure they are completely dry before you put them away.

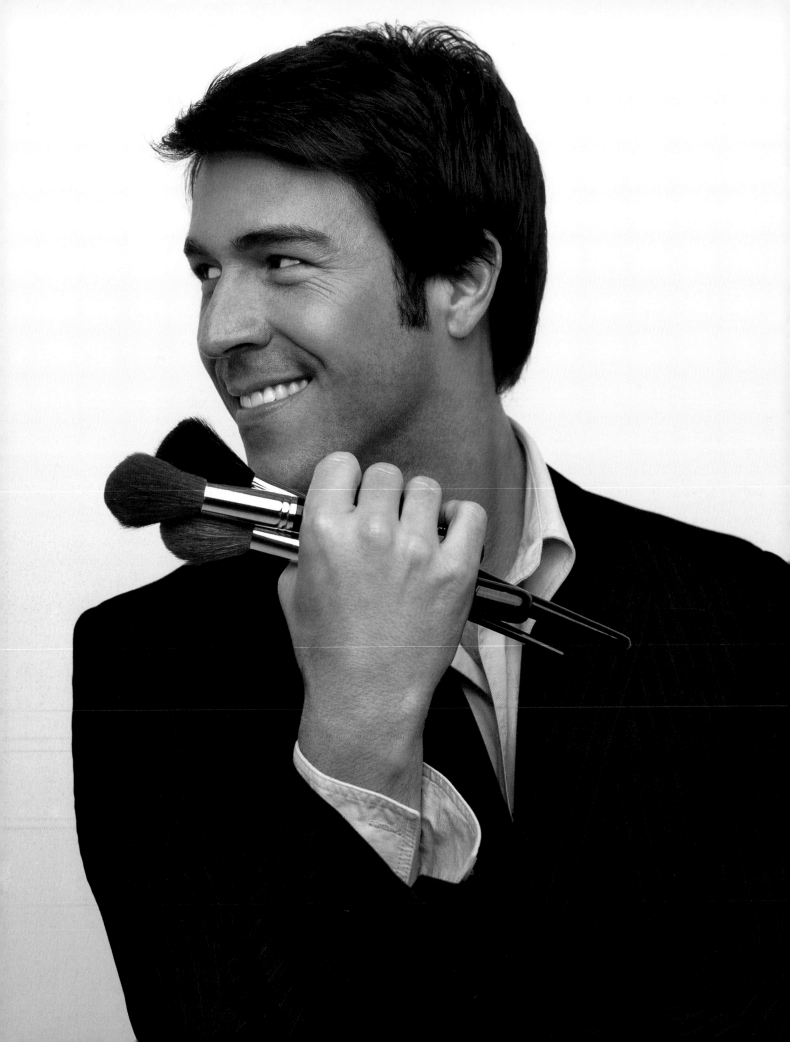

If you're using the tiny brushes that come with powder, blush, or eye shadow, you should upgrade. They're okay in a pinch or to save space in your beauty bag when you're traveling, but that's about it.

find your look

Grab a few magazines and study the pictures inside. Check out the textures of the makeup worn by the women in the photos. Are the products sheer, shimmery, or opaque? Look at the colors. Is there one shade on the eyes and cheeks or multiple hues blended into one another? When you find a look you love, assess the person's features and coloring. The more they match yours, the more closely you'll be able to copy the look. If you and that person have nothing in common physically, it's okay. You can still be influenced and inspired by the colors and the mood of the picture. Styles and colors change with each season, and while you don't need trends to dictate your look, you can use the changes for inspiration.

consider the big picture

Before you start applying your makeup, decide what kind of look you're going for. Are you trying to make a statement, or are you aiming for a more subtle enhancement? Think of your face as a palette that requires an overall color and texture scheme. Do you want a focal point, like bold lips, or something less obvious, like all-over neutral tones? Each element—eyeshadow, liner, blush, lipstick, foundation—should have its own purpose in relation to the others. Know what your mission is, and choose elements that fit in the bigger picture.

Always keep your hair and clothes in mind when planning your makeup.

complexion perfection

Good skincare and great-looking makeup go hand in hand. If you have a skincare problem, don't expect your makeup or solve it. Make sure you're following a thorough and consistent skincare routine (see pages 58–59).

beauty buddy

Bring a friend when you shop for makeup. Make sure it's someone who will give you an honest opinion. While a salesperson may recommend a color that looks great on you, your beauty buddy can really tell if it's "you" or not.

kyanism

Do It Right Allow enough time for proper makeup application. Do it properly in a well-lit space before leaving the house. Don't do it in your car at a red light or sitting on the bus on your way to work. You'll never look as good as you could if you do your face on the run. (Besides, it's fine to touch up your lipstick and powder throughout the day; it's tacky to do your full routine in front of strangers.)

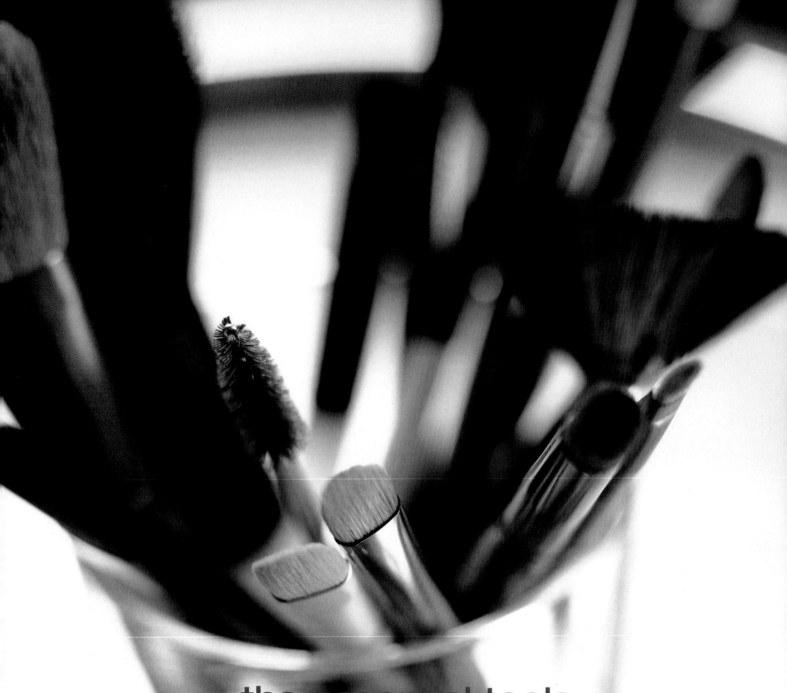

the essential tools

These 10 tools make it easy to put makeup on—and take it off.

Large powder brush • Large blush brush • Eyeshadow brush •

Foundation brush • Velour powder puff • Eyelash curler •

Makeup remover • Cotton swabs • Cotton pads • Tissues

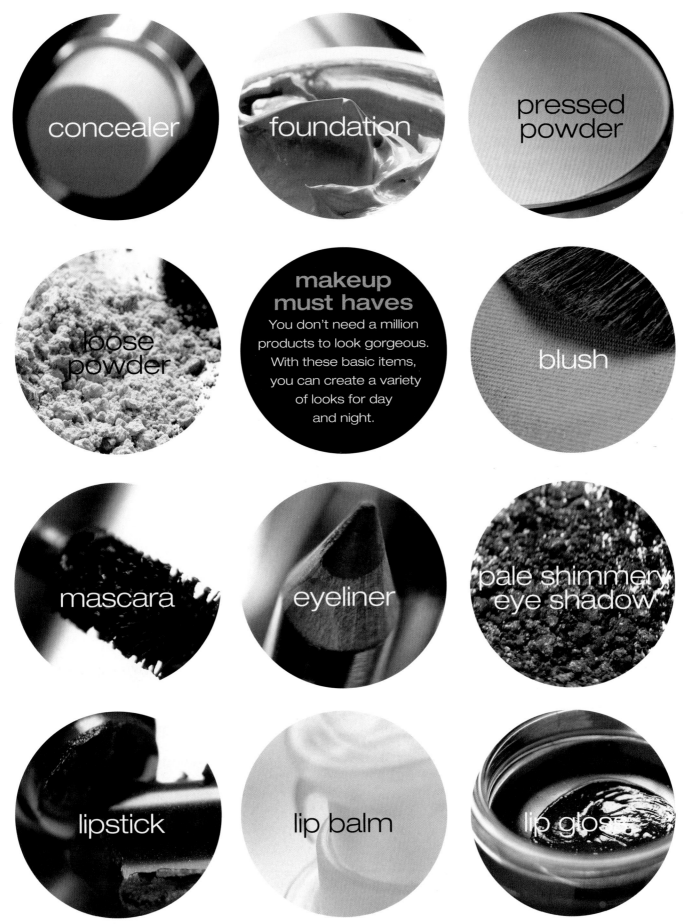

concealer

foundation

pressed powder

loose powder

makeup must haves
You don't need a million products to look gorgeous. With these basic items, you can create a variety of looks for day and night.

blush

mascara

eyeliner

pale shimmery eye shadow

lipstick

lip balm

lip gloss

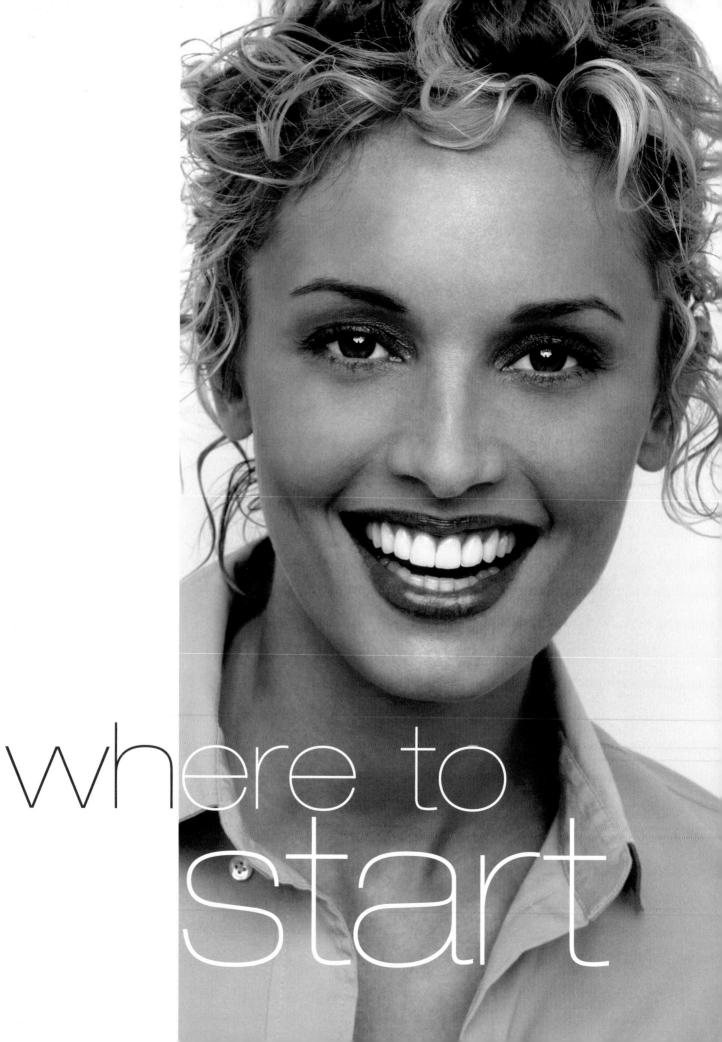

where to
start

In this chapter, I urge you to experiment with color and try various combinations to see if they'll work for you. But before we begin with the essential beauty elements, you'll need to assess your skin tone and see if you have warm or cool coloring. Basically, if your skin has golden undertones, then you're warm; if it has pink undertones, you're cool. (If you sunburn easily, then you're probably cool. If you tan easily, then you're probably warm.) Cool tones are generally better-suited for makeup that is blue-based, such as fuchsia, silver, or lavender. Warm tones generally work well with yellow-based makeup, like peach and gold.

However, combining warm and cool colors is a great way of getting around these "rules." If you have a warm skin tone, you can wear cooler shades; just be sure to combine the cooler shade with a warmer one. Try lavender eye shadow with brown liner, or even a peach shadow with a purple eyeliner. This goes for lipstick too—you can get away with pinker lipstick by applying a gold or warm-toned gloss over it, or a more neutral lip liner underneath.

Foundation, concealer, and powder are the basic makeup products that even out your tone and texture to help your skin look better. Whether you need one or all three depends on your skin and your preferences.

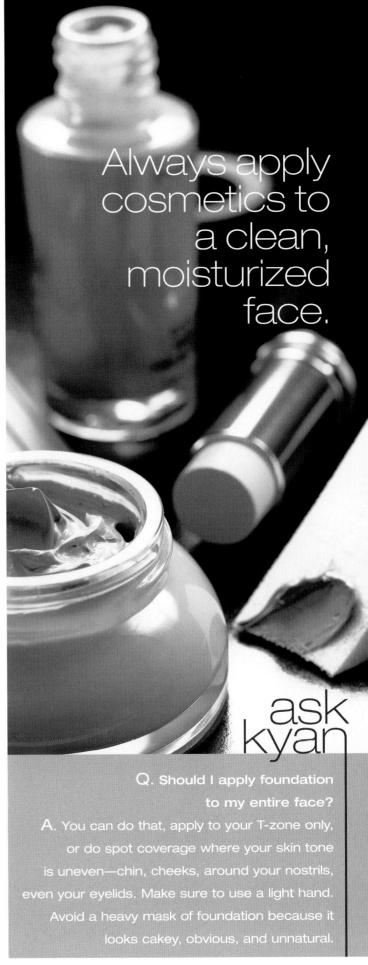

Always apply cosmetics to a clean, moisturized face.

ask kyan

Q. Should I apply foundation to my entire face?

A. You can do that, apply to your T-zone only, or do spot coverage where your skin tone is uneven—chin, cheeks, around your nostrils, even your eyelids. Make sure to use a light hand. Avoid a heavy mask of foundation because it looks cakey, obvious, and unnatural.

foundation

This is a terrific product for evening out your skin tone. It comes in a variety of formulations.

liquid foundation

The most common type of foundation, this provides heavy, medium, or sheer coverage. (Sheer is the most natural-looking option and will feel the lightest on your face.) Liquid formulas contain lots of extras these days. There are options for oily, dry, and combination skin, and ones for anti-aging and radiance boosting. You also can choose a specific texture, like dewy or matte (which means shine-free).

compact foundation

This provides sheer or medium to heavy coverage. The sheer version generally has a gelatin-like texture and comes in an airtight container. The heavier one is the consistency of concealer.

stick foundation

This provides the heaviest coverage and can double as concealer.

how to apply foundation

- A foundation brush is my favorite when I'm getting made up for a photo shoot. Also, it's the most sanitary option, because your fingers don't touch the product or your face.
- A cosmetics sponge is another option. Use dry, or you can dampen the sponge slightly to get a sheer application. (If you reuse your sponges, wash them regularly!)
- Your fingers are a perfectly acceptable option, as long as they're clean.

the perfect match

Just as you have to kiss a lot of frogs before you find your prince, you have to sample a lot of shades before you find the right foundation. If you're shopping somewhere that lets you try before you buy, narrow your search to three colors, then put a stripe of each on your makeup-free face, right under your cheek. Don't try the colors on the back of your hand. You won't get the same results. Blend each color into your skin a tiny bit, then head for natural light. If necessary, ask the salesperson for a mirror you can carry to the nearest window. The color that disappears into your skin is the ideal shade for you.

Pay attention to the underlying tones of your foundation. Make sure you don't pick a shade that's too pink or too yellow for your skin.

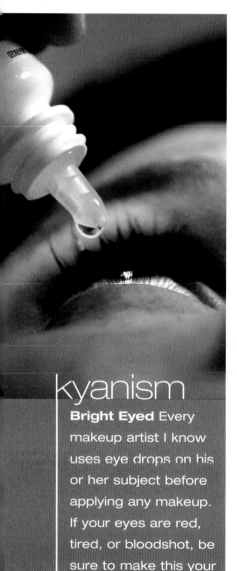

kyanism

Bright Eyed Every makeup artist I know uses eye drops on his or her subject before applying any makeup. If your eyes are red, tired, or bloodshot, be sure to make this your first step.

Always mix in your palm or on the back of your hand. Don't mix in the bottle!

mix master

- If you can't find an exact match, don't despair. Do what makeup artists do and blend two shades together.

- For skin that glows, mix a drop or two of liquid shimmer in your foundation.

- If you're feeling pale, mix in a few drops of liquid bronzer.

- You can use liquid shimmer or liquid bronzer instead of foundation for a daytime spot treatment, or all-over coverage for a nighttime look. A little bit of these products goes a long way, so try mixing several drops of each with a few drops of moisturizing lotion for sheer, easy application.

- I think foundation that looks sheer and natural is the prettiest. If your foundation provides too much coverage, mix in a few drops of moisturizing lotion to dilute it.

kyanism

Eye on the Prize
Remember the goal? You want people to see *you* when they look at your face, not a layer of makeup. If you don't need or like foundation, skip it entirely and apply concealer on top of your clean, moisturized skin wherever needed.

concealer

If I had to pick my favorite makeup product, it would be concealer—or "bag be gone," as I like to call it. When I get to the set, I always ask for a little "bag be gone," lip balm, and eye drops. The combination helps me look awake and refreshed, no matter how early or late we start shooting.

Concealer generally provides more coverage than foundation and is used for spot coverage of dark circles, redness, and blemishes. Concealer comes in different forms, and the intensity of each product varies.

liquid concealer
This comes in a tube with a wand applicator and provides light coverage.

cream concealer
This comes in a pot, tub, or compact and provides medium to heavy coverage.

stick concealer
This comes in a tube and provides medium to heavy coverage.

under or over?
Some makeup artists apply concealer over foundation because the foundation already provides a certain amount of coverage, meaning you need less concealer (or possibly none). When I'm made up for TV or some event, I like concealer before foundation because it evens out my skin tone more effectively for the close-ups and bright lights. For day-to-day use, apply foundation first and then concealer as needed.

where to apply
To eliminate dark circles, dot concealer inside the bridge of your nose where your eye socket begins and extend under your eye. Apply with your finger or a concealer brush. If you have redness or discoloration under your lower lashes, use a brush to apply a very thin layer of concealer there. Most people forget this area.

Blend well, but be gentle. The skin around your eyes is sensitive to tugging and pulling.

You also can apply concealer to your chin, the area between your brows, and around your nostrils. Just dot on and blend.

kyanism

Finger Tip If you're using your finger to apply foundation or concealer around your eyes, use your ring finger, not your index finger. (And of course, be sure to wash your hands right before applying.) The pad of your ring finger is softer, and it's better for the delicate skin around your eye.

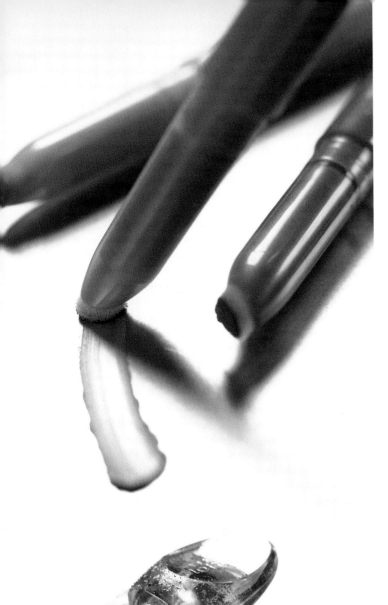

lighten and brighten

Generally, you want a concealer that blends seamlessly with your skin tone, but you can use a lighter shade to brighten your under-eye area. Pick something that's just a hint lighter.

good-bye, pimples

Concealer is a godsend when you've got a few zits to cover. And contrary to popular belief, hiding pimples with makeup does not slow their healing. But if you're concerned about that, there are also medical concealers available today.

Using a brush, dot some concealer onto the blemish. With a very light touch, blend the product away from the pimple so that the concealer disappears into the skin. If you need to give the concealer extra staying power, use a puff to gently dust loose powder on top of the concealer. Just be sure to do this carefully. The end result should look smooth, not cakey. You don't want to draw even more attention to your pimples.

I'd like to use this opportunity to remind you again not to pick at your pimples. (See pages 64–65). It's hard to hide your zits with concealer when they're scabby or raw.

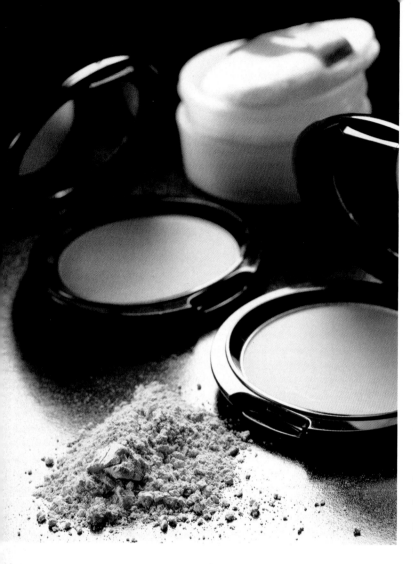

powder

This is the finishing touch for any look. Wear it over your foundation and concealer to set your makeup or reduce shine, or wear it alone over clean, moisturized skin. Some powders are labeled as translucent, which means they won't add color to your skin, but people with darker skin tones might find them too ashy. Other powders come in a variety of complexion colors. Shimmer powders have a bit of pearl or sparkle to give your face a glow. All powders, except shimmery ones, will give you a matte, shine-free face.

loose powder
This is a formula that's been ground into extremely fine particles, similar to baby powder. It comes in a tub or box and is best applied with a puff or a big brush. Loose powder can be messy to deal with and it's easy to apply too much. Before touching your face with a puff, shake off the excess product. Using a brush? Tap it against your sink or another hard surface to remove the excess. Apply over your entire face using a light touch.

pressed powder
This is loose powder that's been pressed into a solid cake. It comes in a compact with a puff. Because it's so portable, you can toss it in your bag and use it for touchups throughout the day. The puff can become dirty quickly, so wash or replace it regularly.

bronzer
This comes in cream, liquid, gel, or powder form and can be used to mimic a sun-kissed look—not an overall tan. Use a foundation brush, sponge, fingers, or powder brush and apply wherever the sun would hit your skin: forehead, nose, cheeks, chin, collarbones, and shoulders.

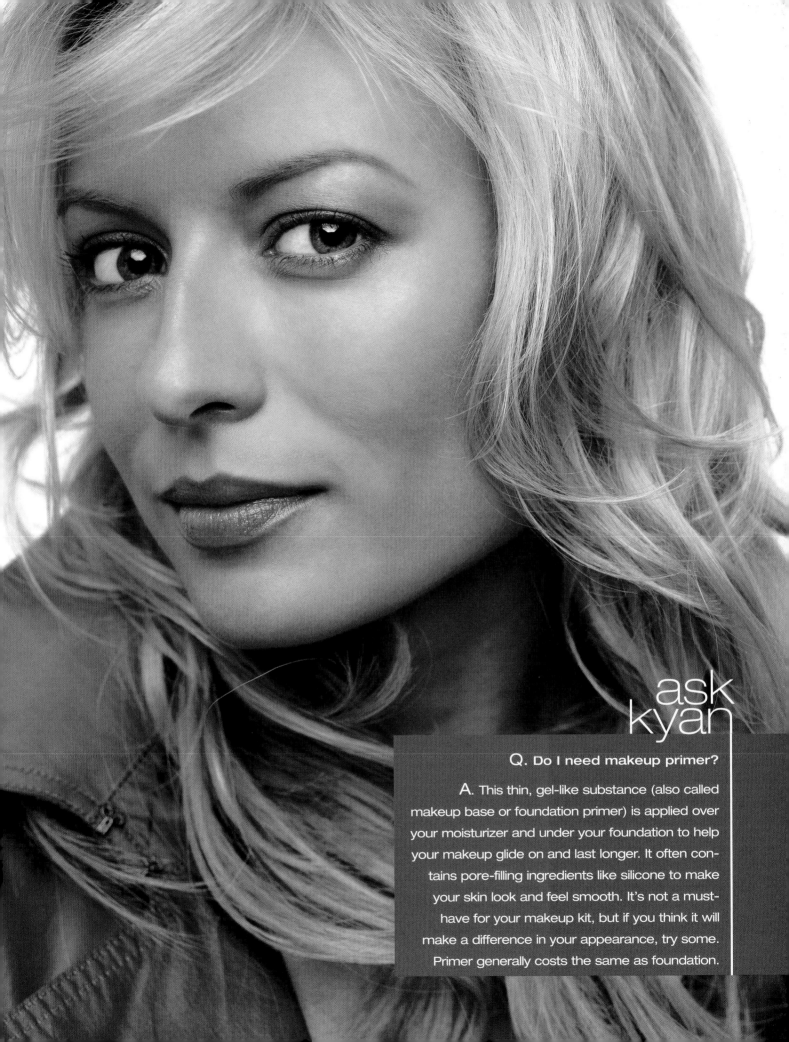

ask
kyan

Q. Do I need makeup primer?

A. This thin, gel-like substance (also called makeup base or foundation primer) is applied over your moisturizer and under your foundation to help your makeup glide on and last longer. It often contains pore-filling ingredients like silicone to make your skin look and feel smooth. It's not a must-have for your makeup kit, but if you think it will make a difference in your appearance, try some. Primer generally costs the same as foundation.

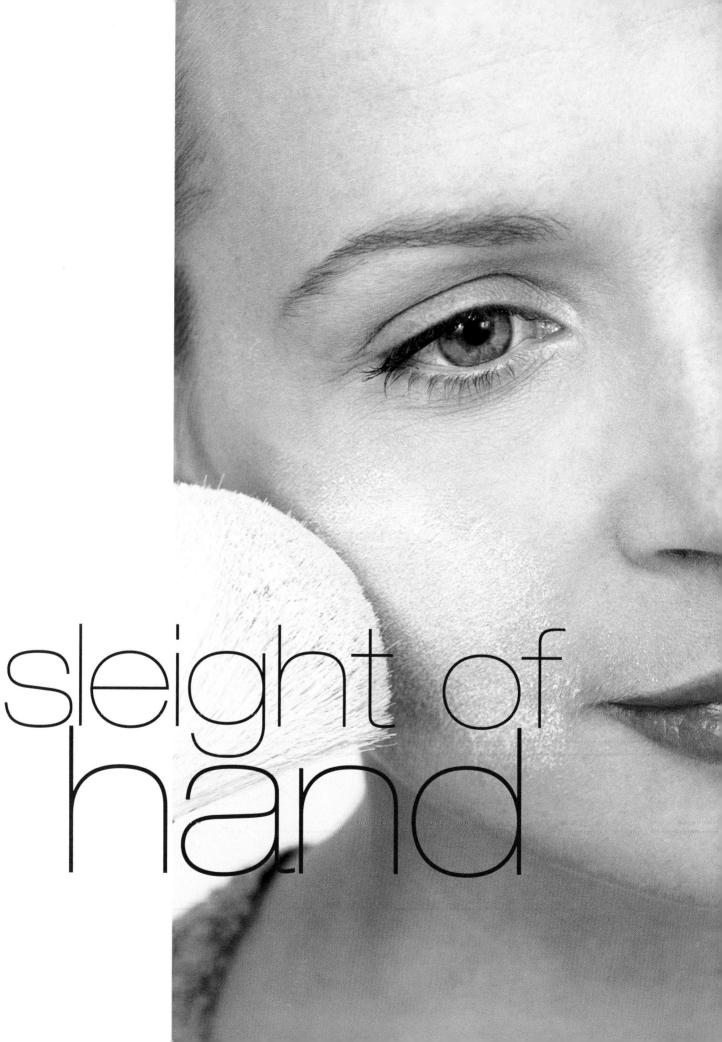

sleight of
hand

Now's a great time to discuss using makeup to play up or play down certain features. Contouring is the use of dark colors to set features back, or make them appear smaller or less obvious. Highlighting, on the other hand, is the use of light colors to emphasize features or make them pop.

For the contouring tricks listed below, you can use bronzer, dark powder, or eyeshadow. The product should be in the taupe or brown family and be a few shades darker than your skin tone. All of these tricks require a fair amount of skill, plenty of practice, and a lot of blending! You're trying to fool people's eyes, so you shouldn't see any obvious lines when you're finished.

contouring tricks

slim down your nose. Apply a stripe of color down each side of your nose and around the tip. Avoid the strip that runs down the center of your nose.

strengthen your chin. Apply contouring product along your jawline.

create cleavage. If you're wearing something low cut, apply a little contouring product up and down the area right between your breasts.

getting cheeky

The one product that can make you look sexy, pretty, and healthy in an instant? Blush. Everybody looks better with a little flush to her cheeks and there are different ways to get that look.

powder blush The most basic and popular kind of blush, this is available in dozens of colors and textures. Don't be afraid of buying bright, vivid shades. These generally appear much lighter when applied. The most natural looking blush is the same color that you flush when slightly exercised. Powder blush is best applied with a large blush brush. Remember to remove excess product by tapping the brush against your sink or another hard surface. If you've applied too much or need to blend, use a velour powder puff.

cream blush This comes in a pot or as a stick and is perfect for dry or mature skin types, but it shouldn't be used on top of powdered skin. Apply and blend with your fingers or a sponge.

liquid blush Want that flushed schoolgirl look? This is the easiest way to get it, but you'll have to work fast—this formula dries quickly and is hard to blend. The liquid temporarily stains the skin, so use a cotton swab for application to avoid tinted fingertips. Practice a few times before wearing this in public.

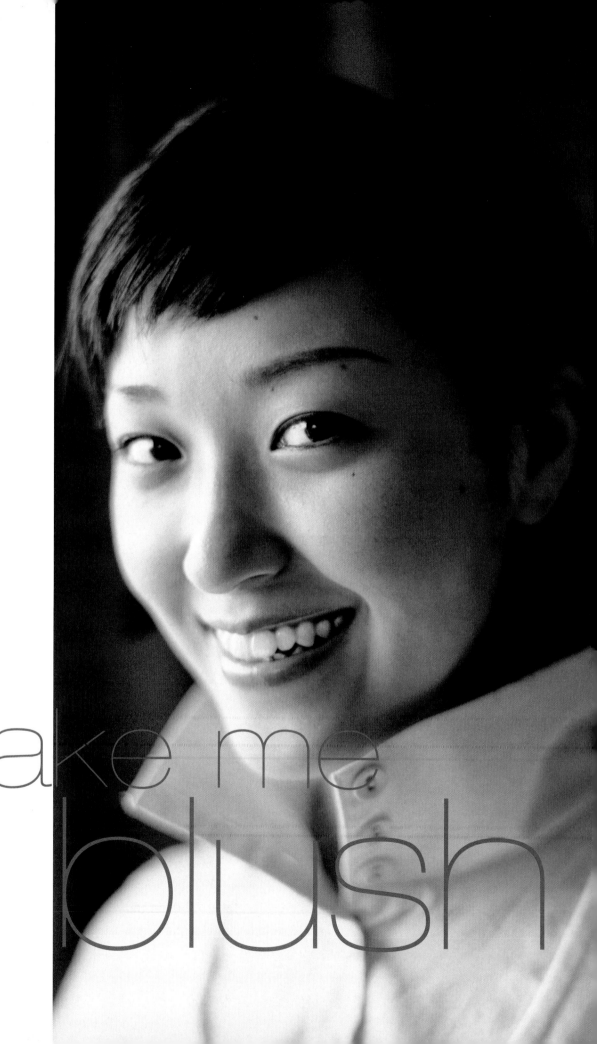

make me
blush

Flushed and healthy are the buzzwords I want you to keep in mind before you apply any blush, because you'll look prettiest when your makeup appears to be natural. To start, find the apples of your cheeks. These are the fleshiest parts and feel somewhat round when you smile. You can apply your blush here and stop, or you can extend it along your cheekbones to the start of your hairline. Whatever you decide, blend well! A big stripe of blush along your cheekbone is not a great look.

layering

To give your blush dimension and staying power, apply cream blush and blend, then apply powder blush directly on top of that. Blend gently with a velour powder puff.

emphasize your cheekbones

Once you've applied your blush and blended it, take some shimmery powder and apply above your cheekbones and, if you like, all the way to your hairline. Or you can curve the powder in a C shape from the middle of your cheekbones around the outer corners of your eyes to your temples. Blend with your fingers or a velour puff.

define your cheekbones

Apply your blush on the apples of your cheeks and extend along your cheekbones. Take your contouring product or a small amount of neutral blush and, avoiding the apples, apply under your cheekbones to the hairline. Blend. This will create a less round-looking face.

kyanism

The Right Order

Any lotion or cream product, such as concealer, cream blush, shimmer cream, or cream eyeshadow, won't glide over a powdered surface. Always use creamy products before you apply powdery ones, or your skin won't be able to absorb the cream and you'll end up with a messy-looking texture.

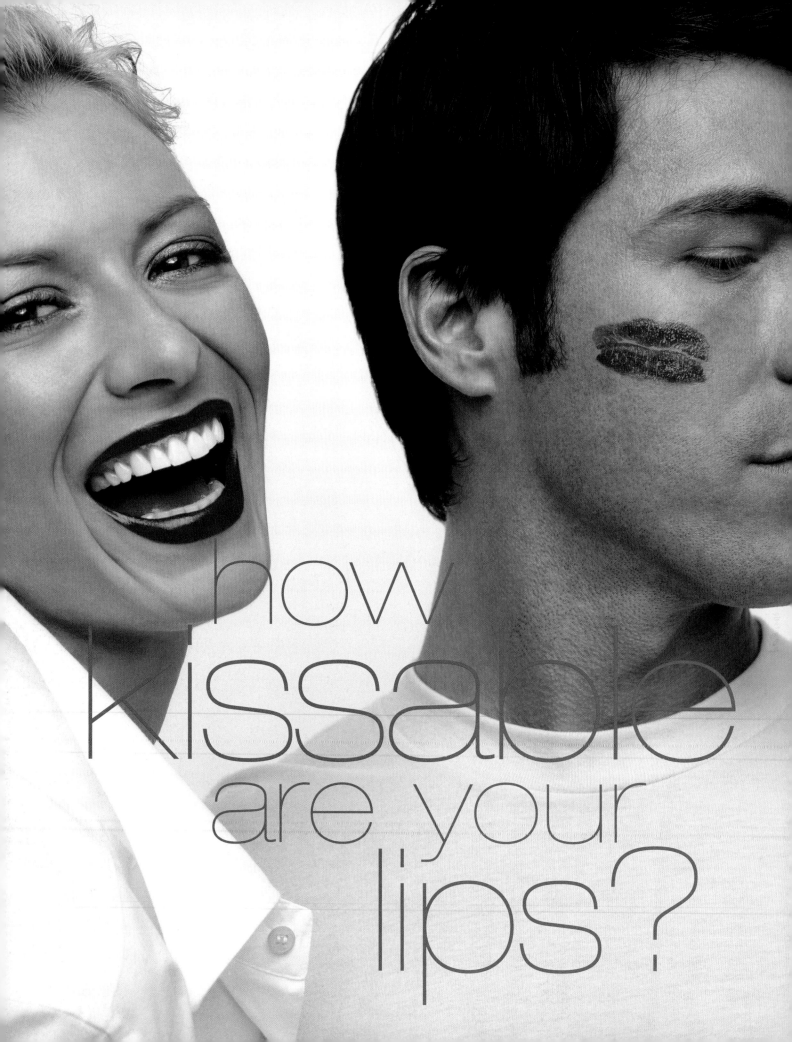

how kissable are your lips?

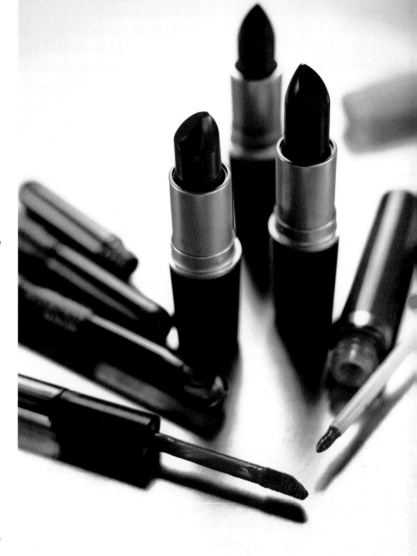

Before you put on lipstick or slick on some gloss, your lips should be in top condition. Color on top of dry, cracked lips? Yuck. We talked about lip maintenance in the previous chapter (page 57), so hopefully yours are soft and flake-free by now. Before applying any makeup, slick on some balm and wait for it to absorb.

You should carry lip balm with you every day. Not that I need to tell you this, but stick lip balm is the best option. It's a lot less germy than a pot of balm into which you (and perhaps your friends) stick your fingers all day long.

lipstick therapy
To me, lipstick seems like one of the great things about being a girl. There's no quicker way to update your look, improve your mood, or pull yourself together. Slick on some color, smack your lips together, and you're on your way. That little ritual makes you feel better every time, doesn't it?

lip look
Finding the right color is the first step. Remember to choose a product in accordance with the rest of your look. If you're making a statement with your eye makeup, your lipstick should play a secondary role.

Scarlet, berry, burgundy, and other rich shades can look sexy, edgy, or classic, depending on your style and your attitude. Just remember that these high-maintenance colors require frequent touch-ups throughout the day.

Be sure to test various shades of a particular color. You may not look great in an orange-red, for example, but a blue-red could be fabulous on you.

make it last
Here's the old-fashioned way to make your lip product last: After you apply your lipstick, blot your lips against a tissue (don't use the super-soft kind or you'll get fuzz all over your lips), then dust a tiny bit of loose powder over your lips. Reapply your lipstick, blot again, and you're good to go.

kyanism

Germ Alert If you want to sample lipstick before you buy it, try the product on the back of your hands. If you really want to see how it looks on your lips, ask the salesperson to remove the top layer for you. (They should have a lipstick-slashing tool on hand —I often had to do this when I worked at a beauty boutique in New York.)

Applying lip liner first will give your lipstick extra staying power. Fill in your entire lip area. Just outlining your lips won't help your lipstick last and will leave you with an obvious outline if your lipstick wears away.

You also can try a long-wearing lipstick. In the past, these were terrible products that dried out your lips. Today, they're so much better because companies have dramatically improved the formulas and they are actually moisturizing. Most long-wearing lipsticks consist of two products: a liquid lipstick and a balm or gloss. Apply the liquid to naked lips, let it dry completely (this step is important!), then slick on the balm or gloss. Reapply the gloss throughout the day to keep your lips moist. The best of these products can last eight hours or longer.

Another long-lasting option is lip stain. Some come in marker-shaped applicators, others come in little bottles of heavily tinted liquid. If yours comes without an applicator, use a cotton swab rather than your fingers. Be sure to apply balm throughout the day because stains can be very drying.

ask kyan

Q. I always seem to get lipstick on my teeth. What can I do about this?

A. Once you've applied your lipstick or gloss, place your pinky finger in the center of your mouth, close your mouth around your finger, then pull out your finger. This will remove any product that would have wound up on your teeth.

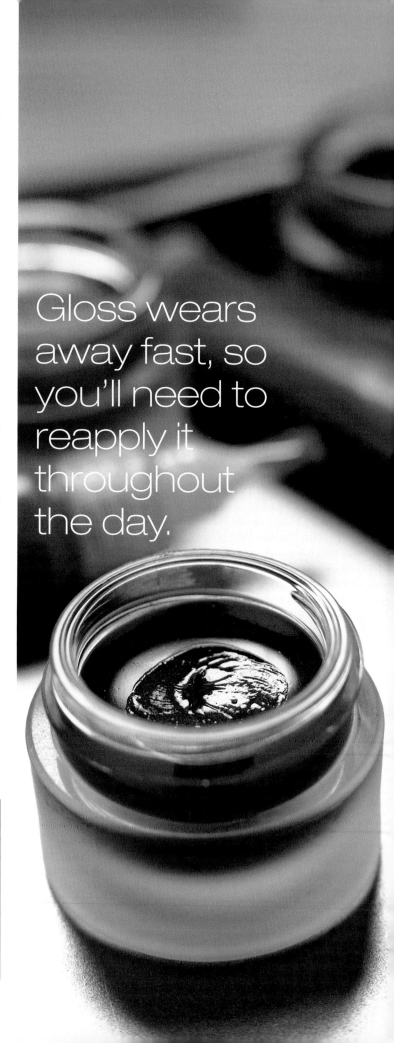

Gloss wears away fast, so you'll need to reapply it throughout the day.

go for the gloss
Nothing's sexier than lip gloss, but a little goes a long way. You don't want goopy lips, especially if you have hair that's chin length or longer. Any wind and forget it—you've got a mouthful of hair.

lip tricks

about pout
After you've applied your lipstick or lip gloss, put a dot of concealer, white eye shadow, or pale shimmery gloss (whatever you use should be paler than the base lip color you're wearing) right in the center of your lower lip. Blend slightly. This will add dimension to your lips.

playing cupid
After you've applied all your lip products, take a white pencil, concealer, or shadow and trace along the cupid's bow (the middle-third area) of your top lip. Again, blend slightly. This gives the illusion of fuller lips.

fill 'em up
Want to make your lips look bigger? Use a lip-colored liner and trace right outside your entire lip line. Don't exaggerate the line too much, or your lips will look messy and cheap. Apply lipstick or gloss on top of that, but stick to light or medium colors.

Wondering about those lip-plumping products? Don't waste your money. Most don't work and those that do only work temporarily.

shrink 'em down
Want to make big lips look smaller? Trace just inside your lip line with a skin-colored pencil. Apply your lipstick or gloss inside the line, using a lip brush for precision.

Dark lipstick and gloss make small lips look smaller, but they call attention to big lips.

kyanism

Lose the Liner!
This is my biggest beauty don't—dark liner with a lighter-colored lipstick in the center. Where did this look come from? If you're a guilty party, engage in a little beauty rehab and break the habit.

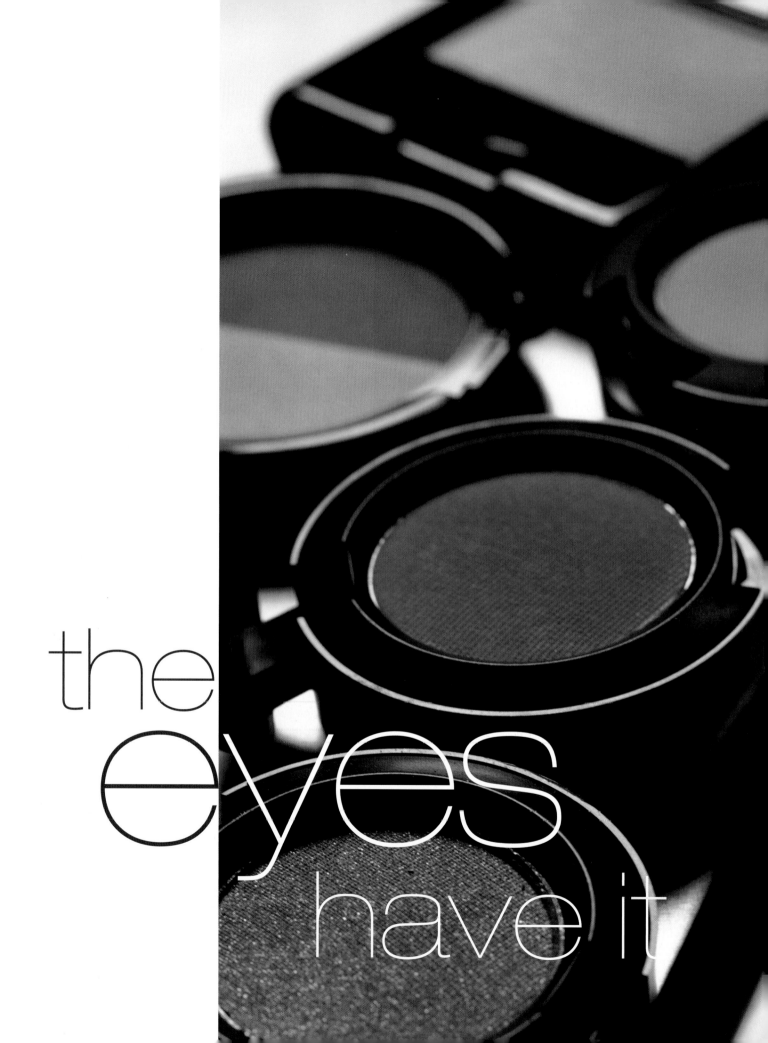

the eyes have it

When it comes to eye makeup, it

helps if you understand your eye shape. When you look in the mirror, do you see a lot of eyelid from your upper lash line to your brows? Or do you see very little? Is the center crease of your lid visible?

In the first case, you can do a lot more with your shadow and liner because you literally have a bigger canvas. You can do the classic contoured look, where you color your eyelid with a medium-toned shadow, highlight your brow bone with a pale shade, and brush a dark contour shadow along the crease of your lid. If your eyes are close together, don't extend the contour color the entire length of the crease. Do the outer half only. This technique will make your eyes look like they're farther apart.

If you don't have much visible eyelid, you can do a modified contour, where the darker color is applied from the lash line to right above the crease, which you can't see when your eyes are open. Skip the medium-toned shade and use a pale shade along the brow bone.

When you apply the shadow to the crease, keep your eyes open and look straight ahead at the mirror, applying the shade just above the actual crease. If you close your eye while applying on the crease, the shadow will just disappear when you open your eye.

beauty bargain When buying eyeshadow,

select compacts that contain several shades and textures within a color family. They'll allow you to experiment with tricks that single colors just won't, and it's great value because you get so many options.

the simple sweep The easiest look to pull

off is one shadow brushed across your entire eyelid, from your lash line to your brow bone. You can do this with any color, but I love how it looks with a light, shimmery tone.

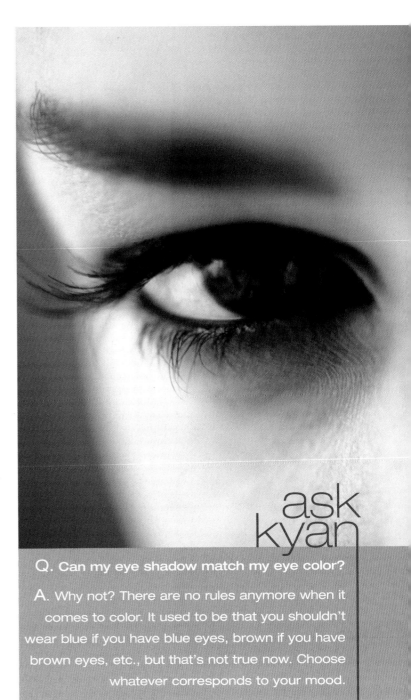

ask kyan

Q. Can my eye shadow match my eye color?

A. Why not? There are no rules anymore when it comes to color. It used to be that you shouldn't wear blue if you have blue eyes, brown if you have brown eyes, etc., but that's not true now. Choose whatever corresponds to your mood.

line and define

The perfect tool for making your eyes really pop, eyeliner comes in pencil and liquid form. Pencil eyeliner allows for more control, and mistakes are easier to fix (since they can be smudged away), so pencils are the smart choice for beginners or if you need to do your makeup fast. Liquid liner creates a cleaner line, but takes a very precise hand to do well because it dries quickly, and once it does, it can be removed only with water or makeup remover.

Here are a few different things you can do with eyeliner:

- Line right along your top lash with a dark color. Smudge slightly with a cotton swab or your finger. Leave the bottom eyelid unlined.

- You can do the same with liquid liner, but don't smudge the line. Using liquid liner takes practice, so don't get discouraged if your handiwork is messy the first few times.

- Try lining your eyes with a pale pencil, like light blue, green, or violet, for a completely different look.

- If your eyes turn down slightly, line along the center third of your top and bottom lashes.

- For a dramatic nighttime look, line around your entire eye and the inside rim of your lower lashes. Work the pencil into the spaces between your lashes to fill any bare spots. Smudge the color slightly with a cotton swab or your finger. (I don't love this look for daytime. It's a little dramatic, and It can make you seem like you're trying too hard.)

- Trace your liner with matching eye shadow for staying power and added dimension.

- Line around your entire eye with sheer, shimmery eye shadow.

- Brighten your eyes by tracing a V shape around the inner corners with a pale, shimmery pencil.

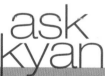

ask
kyan

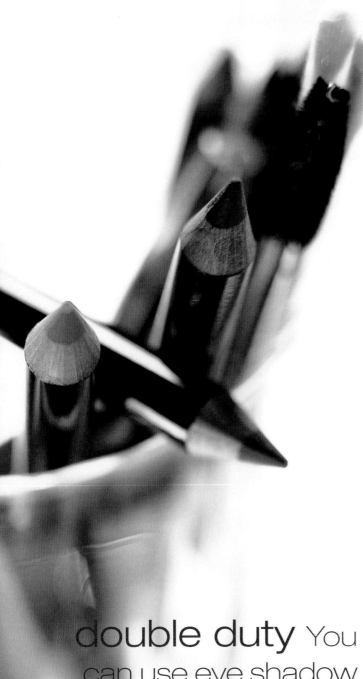

fringe benefits

Long, flirty lashes really wake up your face. First, you have to find the right mascara. There are dozens on the market and it will take a little testing to discover the one that gives you the best results. You need to decide what formula, brush, and color you want. Some mascaras are designed to lengthen, others to volumize, and still others to multiply lashes. Pinpoint the area that needs the most help. Do you want your lashes to be longer? Darker? Once you've narrowed it down, explore the possibilities.

how to apply

Sweep on one coat of mascara from root to tip and let dry. If you need another coat or two, go ahead; just let the mascara dry between each application. For extra volume, apply mascara to the back of your lashes as well as the front.

lash flash

Avoid clumpy lashes. If your mascara wand has too much product on it, wipe it with a tissue before applying. Unless you have very light lashes, don't put mascara on your lower lashes. It never looks natural and it's prone to smudging.

don't share!

There's no quicker way to get an eye infection than by sharing your eye makeup. Your mascara, liner, and shadow should be used by you and you only.

Warning! If you're using a metal eyelash curler, make sure the foam part is intact and in place. I have a friend who chopped off the lashes on one eye because the foam piece was missing and she didn't notice.

double duty

You can use eye shadow as liner by using a thin eye shadow or liner brush to apply. Wet the brush first, then dip into the shadow for a line that really lasts.

ask kyan

Q. Does makeup go bad?

A. Makeup does expire. If the texture of your product changes or it smells bad, throw it away. Mascara should be replaced every six months.

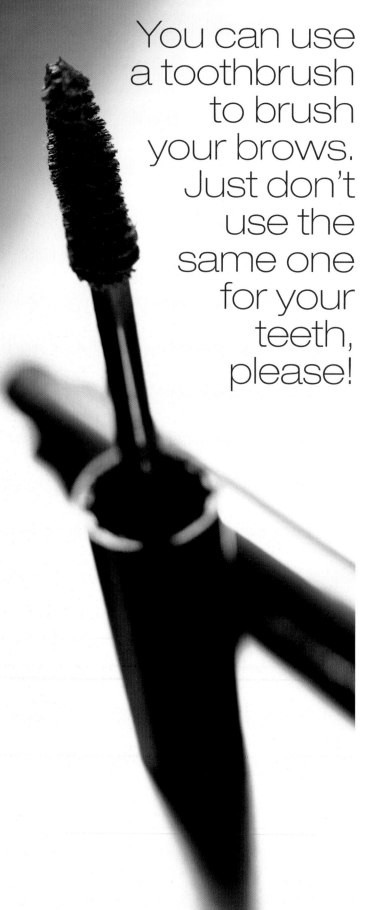

You can use
a toothbrush
to brush
your brows.
Just don't
use the
same one
for your
teeth,
please!

brow know-how Do your

brows need a little love? Whether you've over-
tweezed them (we'll talk about tweezing in the next
chapter) or they're naturally sparse, you can have
the brows you want, thanks to makeup.

First you'll need a few tools. There's a type of
brush that some makeup artists call a spooly. It
looks like a miniature bottle cleaner and it can be
used to comb your brows into place.

Brush your brows upward and into the shape
that you like. Next, take a good look at your brows.
Do they need to be filled in slightly? Do you have
any bald spots? Does the length need to be
extended slightly?

the solutions Eyebrow pencil, eyebrow pow-

der, or eyeshadow. Pick a shade that's lighter than
your brow color; an exact match, especially on
darker hair, will look unnatural.

If you're using powder, apply the color with a flat
brush. You won't be using actual brushstrokes;
rather you'll be applying color by pressing the brush
against your skin. If you're using a pencil, draw with
very slight, feathery strokes. With both methods, do
a little bit at a time and stop to check your handiwork. Clean any mistakes with a cotton swab.

Use this method to fill in the gaps and make
slight fixes, but don't go overboard. Too much
application will be noticeable. You want to stay very
close to your natural brow shape.

If you have brows that need a little grooming, try
one of the brow gels on the market, or use some
hair gel and a spooly brush or toothbrush. Comb
into place and let dry.

day to night

It's easy to take your look from workday to wow:

- Think sexy textures, like glitter, shimmer, or gloss.
- A little glitter goes a long way. If you're wearing some, limit it to one body part or feature.
- Amp up your colors. Think bolder, brighter, darker, or deeper.
- If you wear:

  pinky-brown, try hot pink

  navy, try electric blue

  plum, try bright purple

  taupe, try gold

  black, try silver

- Try a colored mascara. Bright blue, burgundy, and hunter green are fun alternatives to black and brown.
- Powder your face. If you don't normally do this, break out the powder puff for a finished look.

eye way

Whether you're into neutral or neon, your look should always be an expression of your own personal style. Maybe you brush on a little mascara and head out the door, or perhaps you never leave the house without your purple eyeshadow and liner. Realize that your look can change constantly. The more you experiment, the better you'll get at choosing the right products and applying them properly. Anything goes, as long as your personality shines through.

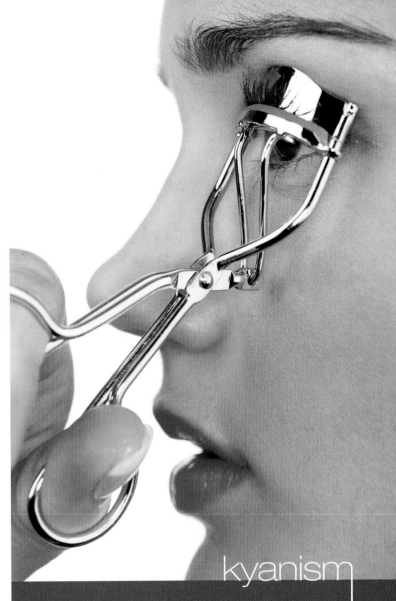

kyanism

Faking It Everyone wants lashes like the ones in ads, but makeup artists use false eyelashes to get those results. If you like that look, try using an eyelash curler before you apply your mascara. I know it looks like a torture device that's going to rip out your eyelashes, but it really makes a difference. Get as close to your upper lash line as possible, squeeze for 5 to 10 seconds, then let go. The idea is to have lashes that curve upward; if your lashes are bent at an angle, you're not using the curler correctly. Make sure the curler hits at the base of your lashes before squeezing.

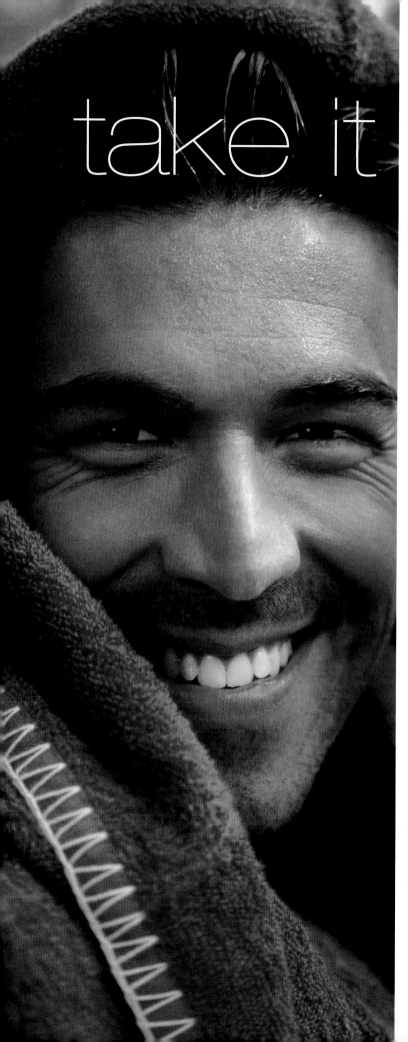

take it off

Sometimes your cleanser is enough

to remove your makeup. Other times, you'll need makeup remover and some cotton pads. If you wear a lot of product, makeup remover wipes are really convenient. Keep them in an airtight container. If they dry out, wet them with a little water.

As we discussed in the skincare section, do not go to bed wearing makeup. This is terrible for your complexion and can lead to clogged pores and acne.

product storage
Applying makeup will be much more enjoyable if your products are well organized. Most places that sell makeup also sell makeup cases. A fun alternative is a tackle box, which you can find at any discount retailer or sporting goods store. You also should have a small makeup bag that fits in your handbag or gym bag, so your favorite products are always within reach.

Wherever you decide to keep your products, make sure it's always clean and tidy. Keep the caps on your lipsticks, don't leave eyeshadow cases open when not in use, and keep your brushes upright and protected so the hair doesn't get mis-shapen. Taking care of your makeup and tools will make them last longer.

the final word

Now that we've talked about all aspects of makeup, let's boil everything down to the essence of what you need to know. I've asked my friend Rudy Miles, a respected makeup artist, to share his favorite advice and beauty mantras. I met Rudy years ago when we worked for the same beauty brand, and since then he's earned a reputation for helping women look their best while letting their true selves shine through.

I wish all of you could have your makeup done by Rudy, but here's the next best thing—his top 10 list:

- Never say never. There are no rules when it comes to makeup. Today, it's all about individuality.

- You need great tools. Most products come with some kind of applicator, but good brushes are a better option.

- Focus on your skin. You need a great skin-care system. Most women talk to me about beauty issues that have more to do with their skin than with their makeup.

- Groom your brows. Don't focus on what's "in" for eyebrows; think about what's appropriate for your face. If you can afford it, have a professional shape your brows.

- Use a good complexion product every day. Whether it's tinted moisturizer, concealer, or powder, find something that addresses the needs of your skin—and that has an SPF 15 or higher.

- Find the perfect blush for your skin type. Powder blush is great for oily skin that needs shine control, while cream blush is ideal for dry skin in need of hydration.

- Treat your lips like your skin. Most women forget this. When you're preparing your skin for makeup, remember this order: cleanser, exfoliator, toner, moisturizer, eye cream, and lip balm. That's a well-prepared face.

- Understand your eye shape. Using certain shades will make your eyes seem bigger, smaller, closer together, or farther apart. Remember, light colors highlight an area, while dark colors can add depth and help you create shape.

- Change your routine. I'm baffled when women tell me they've been wearing the same makeup colors for years.

- Don't strive for perfection. There's natural beauty in imperfection. Try to look your best and accept that as your ultimate form of beauty.

ask kyan

Q. How much makeup is too much?

A. If people look at your face and all they notice is your makeup, you're wearing too much. Of course, red lips or bright purple eye shadow are going to attract attention, but keep two things in mind. One, balance your look. If you're doing a major lip color, keep your eyes neutral, and vice versa. This will center attention on what really matters—you. Two, own your look. It's great to make a statement with your makeup, just do it with confidence.

groomed
and
gor-
geous

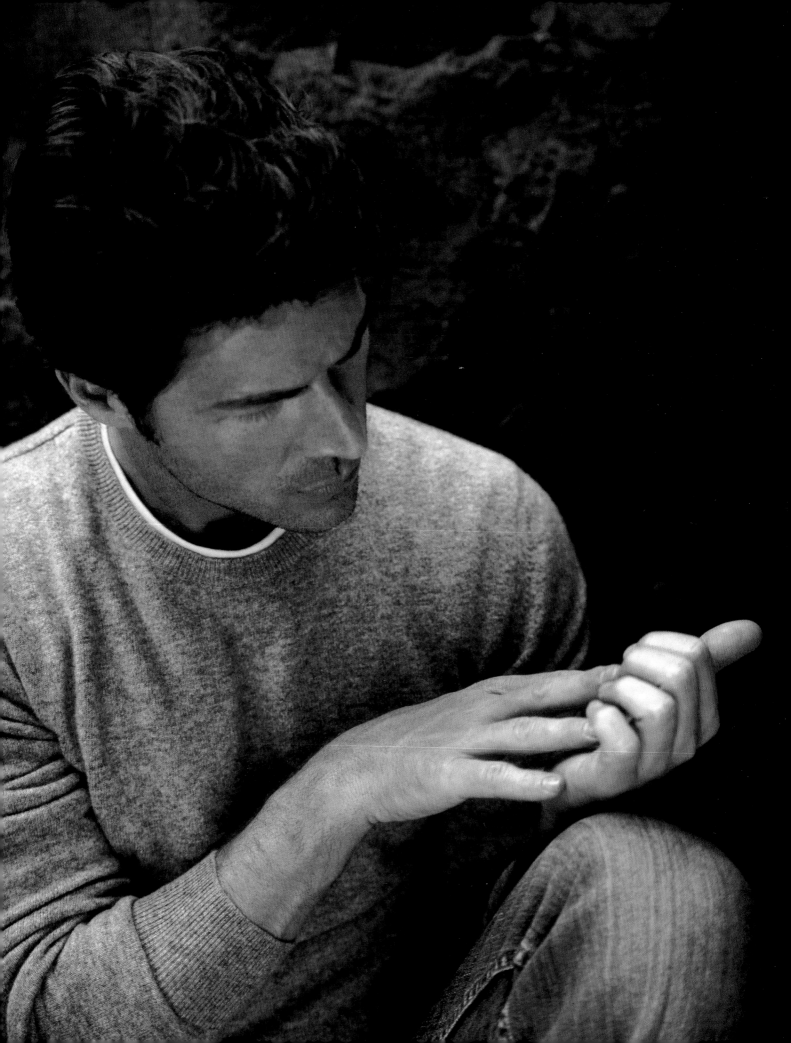

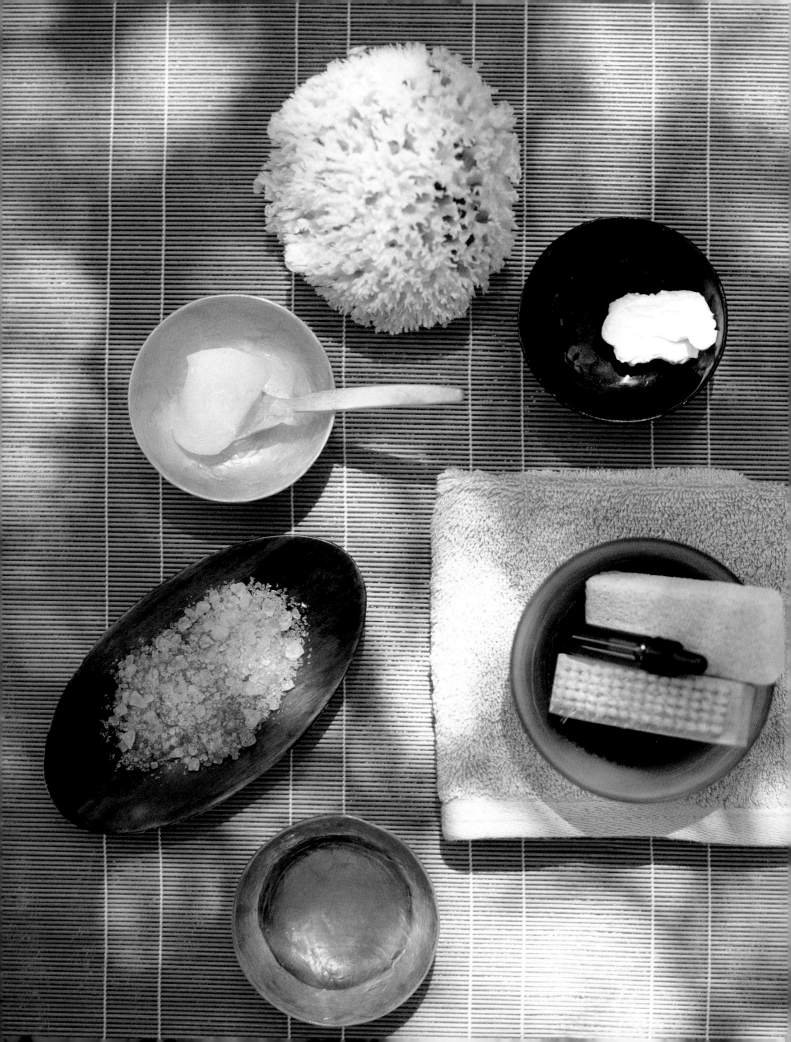

So far, we've concentrated on the basics of beauty—skin, hair, and makeup.
Now we're going to take it a step further and address some other things that contribute to making you the gorgeous creature I know you are.

While you may think that grooming isn't as important as having great skin, hair, and makeup, I'd like to assert that good grooming is essential—simply because it's about the finishing touches that make you feel totally pulled together. What's the point of having glowing skin and fabulous hair if your nails are so yucky that you hide your hands in your lap as much as possible?

On *Queer Eye,* the wives and girlfriends love to complain that their guys are never cleanshaven, their bathrooms are disgusting, or their feet are so gnarly the thought of giving them a foot massage makes their stomachs turn. Does your significant other have any grooming gripes about you? I'm sure you're perfect, but chances are, you've let a few things slip to the wayside. (One of the advantages of dating a straight guy is that he tends not to notice these flaws, particularly if he can't see them in himself!) This chapter shows you how to turn these beauty chores into quick, easy tasks you can actually have fun with.

Grooming may seem like a drag sometimes—who wants to spend 10 minutes shaving their legs when they're late for work? Who feels like staying up late for a last-minute emergency pedicure because there's a sudden heat wave and tomorrow calls for open-toe sandals? You do. It's worth taking the time to try teeth-whitening strips even if no one's ever come out and said you need to (especially if you've been wondering if you should give them a shot). Beautified isn't just about impressing other people—it's about knowing that you're presenting the best possible you. It's also about taking time out for yourself. Follow the instructions in this chapter, and you'll never have to worry about whether you're falling short in any of these areas. Maintain your grooming, and you'll see your strengths—not your weaknesses—when you check your smile in the mirror after lunch. Remember, this is what it means to be beautified.

A lot of the subjects in this chapter can be done in the privacy of your own home, or at a spa or salon. Before we get to the specifics, I'd like to discuss where your grooming will typically take place, and what you can do to enhance your experience there.

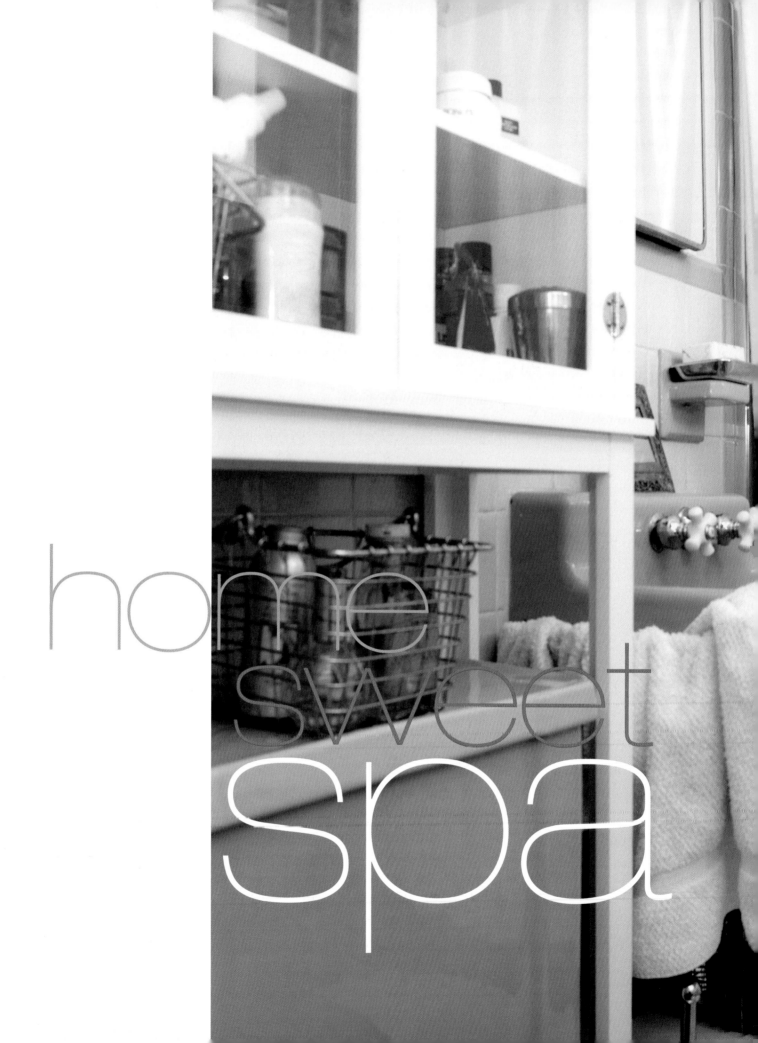

home sweet spa

Everybody has a spa at home. It's called the bathroom. Don't laugh. Your bathroom might look nothing like a spa, especially if you have to share it with your brother, your roommate, your kids, or your kitty's litter box. But from this moment on, I want you to refer to it as "my spa." Has your spa seen better days? Tell yourself and anyone within hearing range that it's slated for renovations. As the spa director, you're responsible for the maintenance of the spa. This means cleaning it yourself or enforcing the rules of the spa: towels get hung on towel racks, toothpaste tubes get squeezed from the bottom up, and the toilet paper roll gets replaced when it's finished.

I know it's not fair that you have to clean up after somebody else, but if you consider the spa your responsibility, you'll be less frustrated by the mess in there. Think of it as straightening up after your spa guests, not the lazy members of your household!

spa renovations

Your spa should be your personal sanctuary. If it needs a good cleaning, get to it. You'll be using your spa for the various grooming techniques introduced in this chapter, so a clean and peaceful atmosphere will set the stage for many pleasant experiences. How inspiring is a grubby bathroom when it's time to shower or floss? Not very. But when you have your own haven, suddenly those tasks don't seem so daunting.

No matter what the mess or problem, from a slow drain to clouded shower-stall glass, there's a product in your supermarket that can solve it.

If the bathroom fixtures are in bad shape, deflect attention away from them with some cosmetic improvements, like a new throw rug or shower curtain.

Is your shower curtain or liner moldy? If so, replace immediately!

Make sure there's a place for your products in the tub or shower. Hang a product organizer in there or get a plastic tote bucket.

Remove everything from the medicine cabinet and evaluate. Toss anything you haven't touched in a year and check expiration dates on any medication.

kyanism

Straight Talk Do you share a bathroom with a straight man? I'll let you in on a little secret. I've seen enough straight men's bathrooms at this point to know that a lot of them don't get the bathroom-hygiene connection. In fact, there's a good chance he'll never get it unless, of course, five gay men show up at his doorstep one day.

You may find that your over-the-counter sinus medication stopped working three years ago.

Short on storage space? Buy a sink skirt or make one with some fabric and Velcro. You'll hide those ugly pipes and have a new place to stash your stuff.

Buy the nicest robe and towels you can afford. They make such a difference. Hang a hook on the back of the door for your robe.

Are any of the walls in bad shape? A fresh coat of paint makes any room look better, and you can hide a multitude of sins with square-shaped mirrors. These come with adhesive backs so you can stick a series of them wherever you like. Mirrors also make small spaces look bigger.

Display fun containers for your cotton swabs, makeup brushes, toothbrush, and toothpaste.

Why not hang some art in your bathroom? Find some cheap flower prints, vintage magazine covers, or old postcards and frame them yourself.

Add a plant (I prefer real ones) and a candle for some glamour.

Buy a small, cheap CD player for your spa tunes.

Install a lock. When the spa is booked, it's booked!

rub a dub Nothing beats a relaxing

bath. You can use any fragranced product you want—bath gel, bubbles, oil, or salts—and just melt away. Personally, I prefer to light a scented candle rather than to add something to the water because my skin is pretty sensitive. If you've got the same problem, try these skin-soothing additions in your bathwater: 1 cup of milk or 2 cups of instant oatmeal wrapped in cheesecloth.

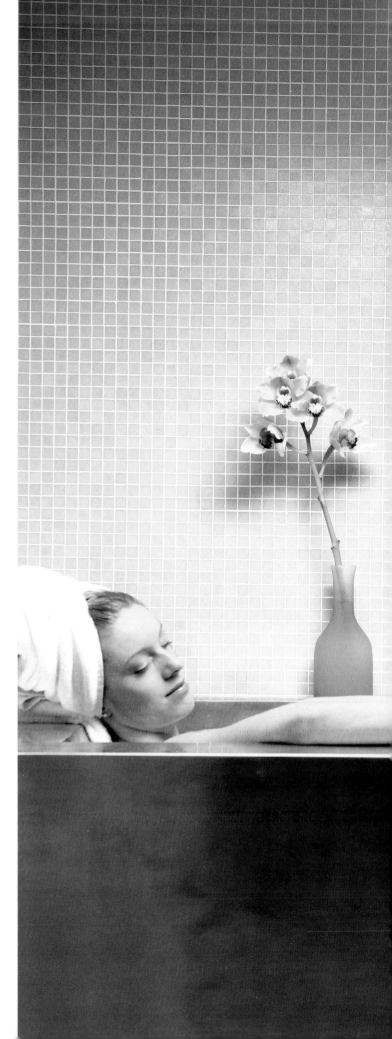

at the salon or spa

As wonderful and convenient as an at-home spa can be, a trip to a salon or spa can be a luxurious, indulgent experience. However, whether you're a regular or a first-timer, it's easy to feel out of place there. Here are a few tips:

don't be intimidated. People get into the spa and salon business because they like making people feel good and look good. If you have questions or concerns (the room's too cold, the music's too loud), speak up. Someone there should be happy to help you. If not, take your business elsewhere.

do arrive early. Show up at least 15 minutes before your appointment, especially if it's your first time. You may have to fill out a questionnaire regarding your health and spa preferences. This also gives you time to enjoy any extras, like the sauna or steam room. Some places have cozy waiting areas filled with magazines, snacks, and beverages. Kick back with your favorite mag and a nice mug of chamomile tea and savor the moment. Being in a relaxed state before your treatment will only enhance the experience.

don't get naked—unless you want to. At most spas, you'll be expected to take off your clothes in a locker room and put on a robe before heading to your treatment. If you don't like getting changed in front of other people, duck into a bathroom stall. There's no reason to feel uncomfortable.

don't bring the bling. Lots of tears have been shed over jewelry lost at spas or left in robe pockets. Spare yourself the headache and the heartache and leave the good stuff at home. If you're heading to the spa after work, put everything in your locker. Do a complete sweep of your locker before leaving.

don't tolerate untidiness. Any spa or salon should be sparkling clean. End of story.

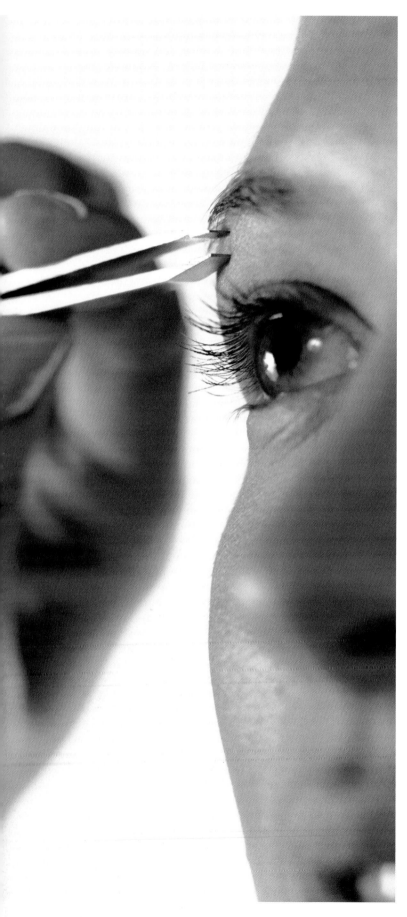

brow wow

Your eyebrows aren't useless little tufts of hair. They frame your eyes and call attention to them, just as a frame does with a painting or photograph. The point isn't to notice the frame—it's to appreciate the artwork. For that to happen, everything needs to be in balance. This means your brows shouldn't be too thick or too thin, and they should have just enough shape and lift to do the job.

the brow virgin

You've never plucked, but you want to start. You can go to a professional, or you can do it yourself. No matter which you choose, it's a good idea to flip through some magazines and study people's brows. See what you like and dislike. Personally, I like brows that look natural but slightly cleaned up. If you go to a pro, be very clear about the shape you want.

The basic idea is to clean up the natural shape of your brows. This means plucking stray hairs and any others that aren't fitting naturally into the overall brow shape. Typically, you should do more work below the brow toward the outer edges and don't do as much with the hairs above it. If you look closely, you'll see that you have your own natural shape that should be embraced, because it most likely complements your face shape. In other words, don't try to create a severe arch if you don't already have much of a natural arch. If you have thick brows, don't tweeze them into a thin line.

The bottom line: Maintenance is key.

A few basic rules to follow:

- Buy a good pair of tweezers. It will make plucking easier and you'll have them forever.
- Tweeze in the direction your hair grows
- Think symmetry. Your brows should match.
- Can't handle the pain? Numb the area with some ice. If that doesn't work, try tweezing after you take a shower.
- It's fine to follow fashion when it comes to shoes, clothes, and handbags, but not your brows. If thin brows are in this season, what will you do next season when bushy brows are back and yours haven't grown back with their usual fullness?
- Unibrows don't look good on men or women.
- When in doubt, see a professional.

do you have a unibrow? If so, start there and remove the hair in between your brows. Never work past the inner corner of each eye. In some cases, you shouldn't even go that far. Pluck one hair at a time, step back, and check your handiwork in the mirror.

where should your brows end? See where they end naturally and keep that length. Just clean up the scraggly little hairs at each end.

the upkeep Your brow hairs will grow in at different speeds, whether you tweeze them or get them waxed. Every few days, tweeze any scraggly, obvious hairs. If you shape them yourself, take a hard look in the mirror every week or so and see if any major work needs to be done.

brow boo-boos

common mistake #1 Plucking too much. Stop now before I take those tweezers away. Brow hair doesn't always grow back. It's temperamental that way.

common mistake #2 The tadpole shape. This happens when the main part of the brow is full and round with a thin little tail trailing behind. Your brows should be nice arches that taper off slightly, not creepy little baby frogs.

kyanism

Arch Rival
Overplucked? Stop tweezing and see if the hairs grow back. If they don't, flip to the makeup chapter and learn how to pencil in your brows. Remember, it's always better to underpluck than overpluck. You can always finish the job later if you decide you want to tweeze more.

good
grooming

razor's edge

Shaving seems like a no-brainer, but when done improperly, it can lead to all sorts of ugly complications. Here are some basic pointers, from someone who has never shaved his legs (or his underarms), but has shaved his face enough to know how to do it best.

- I'm always telling the men on the show to shave "with the grain" because the combination of delicate facial skin and coarse facial hair can result in razor bumps and burns; shaving with the grain is gentler on the skin and will cause less irritation. You don't have to follow this rule when it comes to your legs. The skin on your legs isn't as sensitive and the hair isn't as thick, plus it's nearly impossible to shave with the grain when you're standing in the shower. That said, if you experience razor burn, bumps, or ingrown hairs, try shaving with the grain. You might find the situation improves.

- Shave as often as necessary. Frequent shaving won't cause your hair to grow back thicker or heavier, although stubble definitely feels that way.

- It's a great idea to shave during or after a bath or shower, when the hair is soft.

- You need to lubricate your legs or underarms and soften the hair for the best shave possible. Some women lather up their legs with a bar of soap before shaving, but I don't think that's emollient enough. Women should have shaving products just like men do, such as shaving oil or shaving cream. However, hair conditioner has been known to be a great substitute. It softens hairs and prevents razorburn. Girlfriends of mine who have dark leg and underarm hair swear by this.

- Pay attention. Cuts and nicks tend to happen when you're in a rush.

- Try a razor made for men. They're sharper and more durable than women's because they're designed to stand up to men's coarse facial hair. After using one, you'll toss those flimsy pink things for good.

- Razors with a moveable head, two or three blades, and a lubricating strip are the best.

- Clean the blade after each use and replace before it gets dull. It's time for a new blade when it starts to drag or the lubricating strip is shriveled up.

ask kyan

Q: What do you think about at-home waxing?

A: I try not to think about it. My one and only experience with it was a disaster. I waxed my chest and it was not a pretty sight, because my skin got infected and broke out like crazy. But maybe your skin isn't as sensitive. If you're prepared for the amount of work involved, like heating the wax and dealing with all the strips and the spatulas and the mess, then go for it. Make sure your hands are clean and prep your skin with an astringent first. Afterward, treat your skin with jojoba oil infused with rose, geranium, or chamomile—all are calming to the skin.

armed and ready

It's not a good idea to shave your arm hair. Waxing or laser hair removal is a better option because they don't cause stubble, and stubbly arms are not sexy.

Or, if the hair is dark, consider bleaching it. Buy some cream bleach made especially for body hair at the drugstore. Do a patch test on your inner elbow to make sure your skin's not too sensitive and follow the directions. The product can also bleach your clothes and towels, so be careful.

wax it

This is a great option for your legs, arms, underarms, brows, upper lip, and bikini line. You can do it yourself with kits from your local drugstore, but it's best done by a professional at a spa or a salon. Make sure the waxing area is clean and that any wooden spatulas used to spread wax on your body are new. Once the esthetician is finished, check to make sure he or she didn't miss any spots. If so, politely point them out.

Waxing can hurt like crazy, especially your first time. If you're concerned, take a pill with ibuprofen before your appointment to lessen the pain. Avoid waxing right before or during your period because you're more sensitive then. Also, if you're on Accutane, tell your esthetician because that makes skin more sensitive, too.

mustache be gone

Hair on the upper lip is not a pretty sight, no matter how you look at it. Bleaching is an option for those with a tiny amount of upper lip hair. It can make it look invisible. But if you have dark upper lip hair and lots of it, bleaching won't do the trick; it will leave you with thick peach fuzz. In that case, wax it or consider laser hair removal.

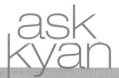

Q. Can I shave my bikini line under any circumstances?

A. You're just asking for ingrown hairs and red bumps. If you're desperate and between waxing or laser appointments, tweezing is your best option. If there's too much hair to pluck and you have to leave for the Caribbean in, say, *five minutes,* go ahead. But just this once. And be sure to use a brand-new razor blade and plenty of shaving cream or gel.

ingrown hairs

These are a total drag. Salicylic acid products help keep them at bay, as does exfoliation with a loofah or scrub. If you have an ingrown hair, you might be able to remove it with a tweezer, but if it's really embedded, see a dermatologist.

laser lesson

Laser hair removal is genius. I had it done on my back a while ago and the results were great. It definitely hurts the first time, but the pain is bearable. It feels like someone is snapping a rubber band against your skin at really close range. The sensation only lasts for a few seconds and lessens with each visit. The sessions tend to take 10 minutes or less, depending on how many body parts you're zapping.

A course of treatment involves three to eight visits, plus annual touch-ups. Why? Because the laser only works on hairs in the active-growth phase, which is why many salons and spas now call it laser hair "reduction" instead of "removal." Some hairs are in the resting and dormant phases and take time to return to the active phase.

The treatment works best on people with dark hair and fair skin because the laser targets melanin, the substance that gives your hair its color. You cannot get a laser treatment if you have tanned skin, but there are other procedures specifically for people with naturally darker skin tones.

Be very careful when getting any kind of laser procedure. Whether you have it done at a doctor's office or a hair-removal center, make sure the person doing the procedure is experienced and well-trained.

As I've mentioned before, don't get laser treatments if you're taking Accutane.

the bikini line

Even though I don't have that strong an opinion about the subject as some guys do—obviously—nicely groomed pubic hair is the way to go as far as I am concerned. I am a firm believer in waxing—not shaving—the bikini line. How far you go is really up to your taste and your partner's preference. If you want to go *au naturel,* so be it. If not, let's talk about your options:

basic bikini wax

This involves removing excess hair and shaping what remains into a neat triangle. It is the least painful and least invasive way to go.

the brazilian

Everything front and back is removed except for a little landing strip of hair. If your bikinis are the teeny variety, this is the one for you.

the full monty

You don't have a hair to spare. Every last bit is waxed away. (And yes, your esthetician gets an eyeful. But you know what? She's seen it all before.)

be dazzled

Who needs boring pubic hair? You can have yours shaped into a heart for Valentine's Day, a thunderbolt for _____ (you fill in the blank), or even initials. If that's not enough, you can embellish the area with adhesive crystals and rhinestones. Tacky? Sexy? Silly? You decide.

hair down there

Let's say you have no interest in waxing, but you want to keep things neat and tidy. Buy a battery-operated bikini trimmer. It's more precise and easier to use than a small scissor. It's a lot easier—and safer—to buzz, buzz than to snip, snip.

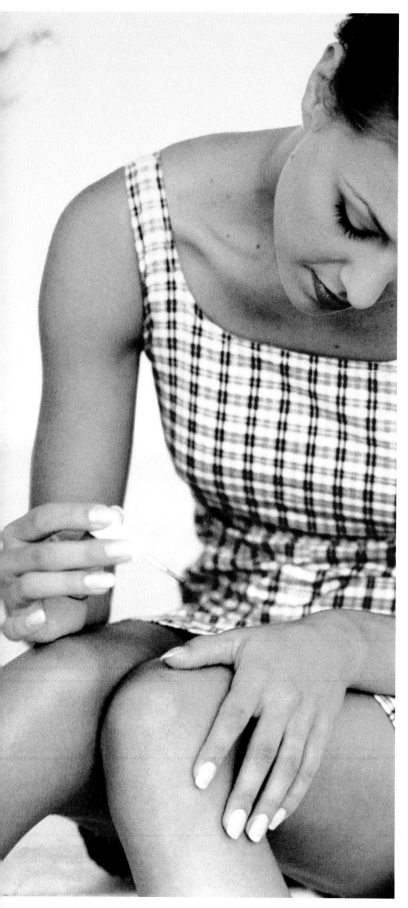

nail
know-how

Let's look at your nails.
Are they pretty and polished? Bitten to the quick? Overgrown and neglected? Whether you realize it or not, your nails say volumes about you. You need to make sure they're communicating the right story to others— and to yourself. It's easy to feel down when your nails are a mess. If you don't know this already, you'll be amazed at how pulled-together you feel when your fingers and toes are neat, clean, and filed to your favorite length.

at the nail salon

If you can spring for a professional manicure or pedicure, that's great. There's something so relaxing about getting your nails done, plus the salon is a great social hub. Go with your girlfriends or your gay boyfriend,* gossip, and have fun. Just make sure that the premises are clean and all the implements are sterilized or disposed of after each use. Don't overlook this in favor of cheap prices. It's no bargain if you get an infection.

*Gay boyfriend (a.k.a. your favorite gay guy). After several months or years of serious commitment, he can be referred to as your gay husband.

When you make your appointment, remember to leave enough time to let your nails dry, and wear open-toed shoes if possible. Nothing ruins a great manicure or pedicure like a smudge. If you have to dash before you're dry, ask your manicurist to apply a quick-dry product.

the perfect manicure
Doing your own nails is easy once you get the hang of it. First, you need the right tools:

Nail polish remover

Cotton balls

Nail clipper or scissors

Nail file

Bowl

Nail brush

Cuticle clipper

Orange stick

Cuticle oil

Hand cream

Nail strengthener

Clear nail polish

Colored nail polish

step 1 Take off any old polish using remover (non-acetone is the least drying) and some cotton balls.

step 2 Decide what length is best for your nails. If yours split, chip, or peel easily, short is best. If you've got a lot of length to lose, clip or trim your nails before filing them. Smooth any rough edges with the file and work into your preferred shape—square, oval, or my favorite, the squoval, a square with slightly rounded edges. When I file my nails, I like to work from the center out to the right side, then go back to the center and out to the left side. Don't file back and forth like you're using a saw. (You've used a saw, right?)

step 3 Fill a bowl with warm water and a few drops of liquid hand soap. You also can include a few drops of essential oil (rose is great) or olive oil. Soak your nails for three minutes. If your nails need a good cleaning, scrub them with the nail brush.

step 4 Wrap some cotton around the orange stick (which is actually not orange, FYI) and gently push back your cuticles. Don't trim each cuticle; instead, use the cuticle clippers to remove hang-nails or ragged bits of skin. Rub a drop of cuticle oil on each nail, then apply hand cream. If your nails are dirty, wrap a tiny bit of cotton around the orange stick and run underneath the tip of your nails. Change the cotton when it gets grimy.

kyanism
Handle with Care
Don't give in to the temptation to pick your hangnails. Soak your fingers in a bowl of warm water with mild soap, and neatly trim the hangnail once it's softened. You can use a nail scissor, but I pre-fer a cuticle clipper. It looks complicated to use, but is easy once you get the hang of it.

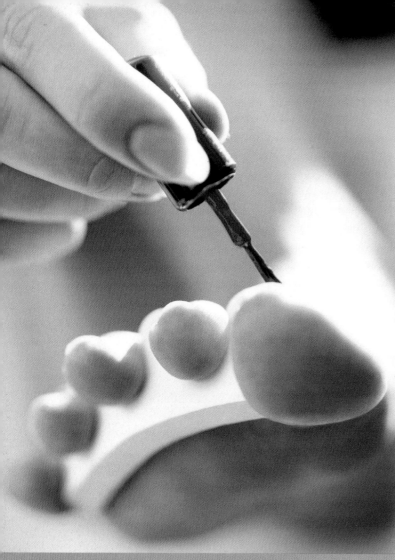

the buff stuff

Too busy to polish your nails? Buffing is a great way to add shine in a snap. Nail buffers are cheap and reusable and are sold in every drugstore or beauty supply store.

fungus factoid

Nail fungus causes discoloration or a softening and weakening of the nails. If fungus is a problem for you, try an over-the-counter treatment or tea tree oil, a natural antibacterial available at most health food stores. If neither works, see a doctor. Don't apply nail polish to a nail that's plagued with fungus. Polish will keep the nail from being able to breathe, and it will enable the fungus to spread.

step 5 Use the polish remover and cotton balls to clean any oil and moisturizer from your nails. This way, the polish will adhere better. If your nails are weak, apply a coat of nail strengthener. If your nails are just fine, apply a coat of clear polish. You don't need a top coat and a base coat. A multipurpose clear polish is just fine. You can stop here if you're a low-maintenance kind of gal, or you can proceed with some color.

step 6 Pick your favorite color and apply one coat. It's hard to paint nails perfectly, so if you've made a mess, wrap a thin layer of cotton around the orange stick or grab a cotton swab and dip into the nail polish remover. Use that to clean up the color. If you happen to have a friend around who can paint the nails on the hand that's difficult to polish precisely, even better.

If you're short on time, you can stop here. Finishing up with a quick coat of clear polish, however, will extend the life of your manicure. Two coats of color topped with clear is even better. Lay low until your nails are dry. Smudged polish is a big bummer.

the softest hands
Many salons offer a skin-softening paraffin treatment in which your hands are submerged in a tub of melted wax, then covered with plastic wrap and fabric mitts. To get similar results at home, wash your hands, then smooth on a really rich hand cream. Put on a pair of cotton gloves (available at most drugstores or beauty supply shops). Wear them while you watch TV or study, or wear them to bed. Leave them on for at least half an hour.

this bites

Gnawing your nails is a tough habit to break, but it sends a bad message. You look like you don't care about grooming, plus you're communicating that you're nervous and unsure about yourself. Chew gum, suck on mints, do anything you can to keep those fingers out of your mouth. Getting your nails polished regularly might help. Who wants a mouthful of nail polish flakes? Yuck. Or keep your nails short. This way there's less to chew.

the perfect pedicure

Basically, you want to follow the same steps outlined in the perfect manicure, but you need a few extra tools and tips.

- Toenails are thicker than fingernails so you might prefer using a nail clipper on them. It's easier to clip toenails once you've soaked them or taken a shower. Let them dry before filing any rough edges.
- Use a foot file before you soak your feet to get rid of any rough, flaky skin.
- Use toe separators, those funny-looking foam things, to keep your toes from touching each other while you polish them. You can use tissues, toilet paper, or cotton balls in a pinch.

sandal season

I have two warm-weather pet peeves:

1. Open-toed shoes with grubby toenails. No time for a pedicure? Wear different shoes.

2. Backless shoes with dry, cracked heels. Moisturize that skin before you leave the house!

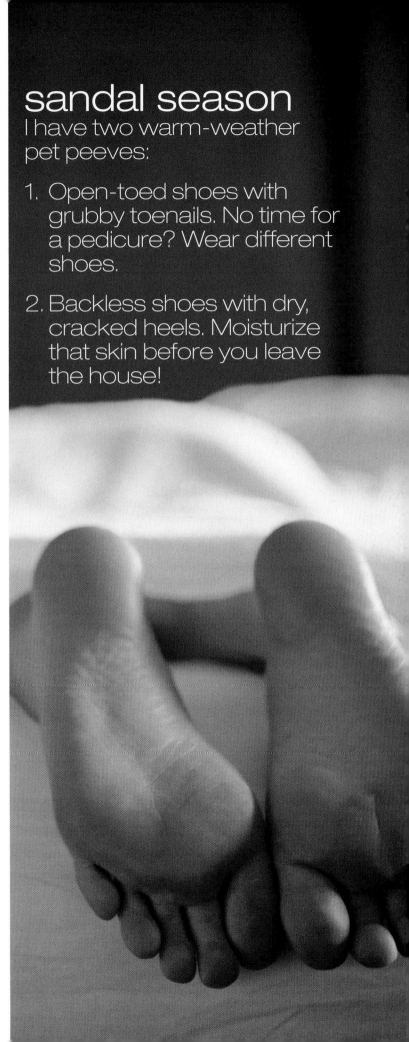

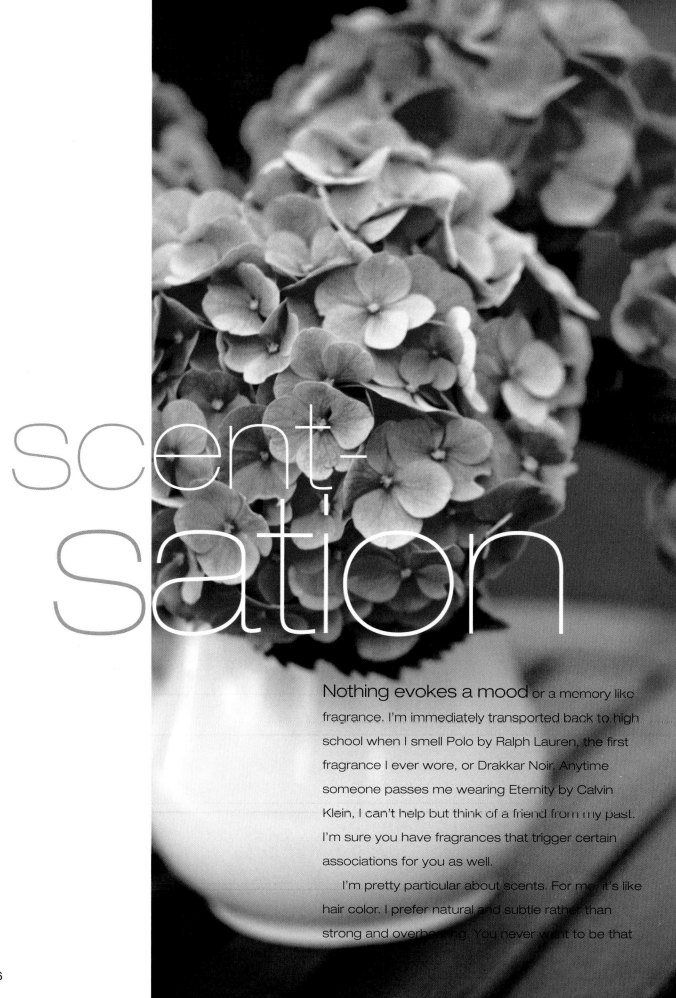

scent-sation

Nothing evokes a mood or a memory like fragrance. I'm immediately transported back to high school when I smell Polo by Ralph Lauren, the first fragrance I ever wore, or Drakkar Noir. Anytime someone passes me wearing Eternity by Calvin Klein, I can't help but think of a friend from my past. I'm sure you have fragrances that trigger certain associations for you as well.

I'm pretty particular about scents. For me, it's like hair color. I prefer natural and subtle rather than strong and overbearing. You never want to be that person who walks into the elevator and over-whelms everyone else with fragrance. In our grand-mothers' era, it was acceptable for your signature scent to waft all around you. Today, it's offputting to wear that much fragrance.

making sense of scent

- Don't wear fragrance to a job interview—unless your job involves fragrance. You want a potential boss to notice you, not your fragrance.
- Don't have a signature scent? That's okay. Mix it up and wear something different every day. You wouldn't wear the same clothes 24/7. Why wear the same fragrance?
- Customize your fragrance. Layer two different scents, or wear your favorite one with a scented oil, like vanilla, clove, cinnamon, or musk.
- Wear oils on their own. I love the blended fragrance oils sold at health food stores.
- A fragrance that smells great on someone else might not smell great on you. Try it first and see how your body chemistry reacts with it.
- Fragrance rarely consists of one scent, like rose or musk. Most are complex combinations of various scents (or notes, as professional perfumers call them). As a result, your fragrance will go through three distinct phases:
  - the top, which you smell as soon as you apply the scent. The top "notes," as they're called, fade quickly.
  - the middle, or heart, which you smell once the fragrance has mellowed a bit.
  - the base, which you smell last. The base notes tend to be the deepest, most sensual part of the fragrance and the longest-lasting.

Because of this, you should try before you buy. Smell how it evolves.

- There are different concentrations of fragrance. Perfume is the strongest (and a little goes a long way), followed by eau de parfum, eau de toilette, cologne, and eau de cologne. (*Eau*, by the way, means "water" in French.)
- Can't smell your fragrance anymore? It's not the scent, it's you. Over time, you can develop resistance to a fragrance. Make sure you don't compensate by wearing too much; instead, try a new fragrance.

perfume for your home

- Use candles to scent your environment. Look for aromatherapy candles made with natural ingredients, as opposed to synthetics, which can be strong and overpowering.
- Don't burn scented candles during a meal. The scent actually interferes with your ability to smell and enjoy your food.
- Skip the synthetic room fresheners and try incense instead. Stick to traditional incense. Fruit-scented incense is always a bad idea.

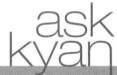

ask kyan

Q. How do I know if I'm wearing too much fragrance?
A. A spritz or two will do. Wear just enough so that a person leaning in for a hug or a kiss gets the faintest whiff and knows how great you smell.

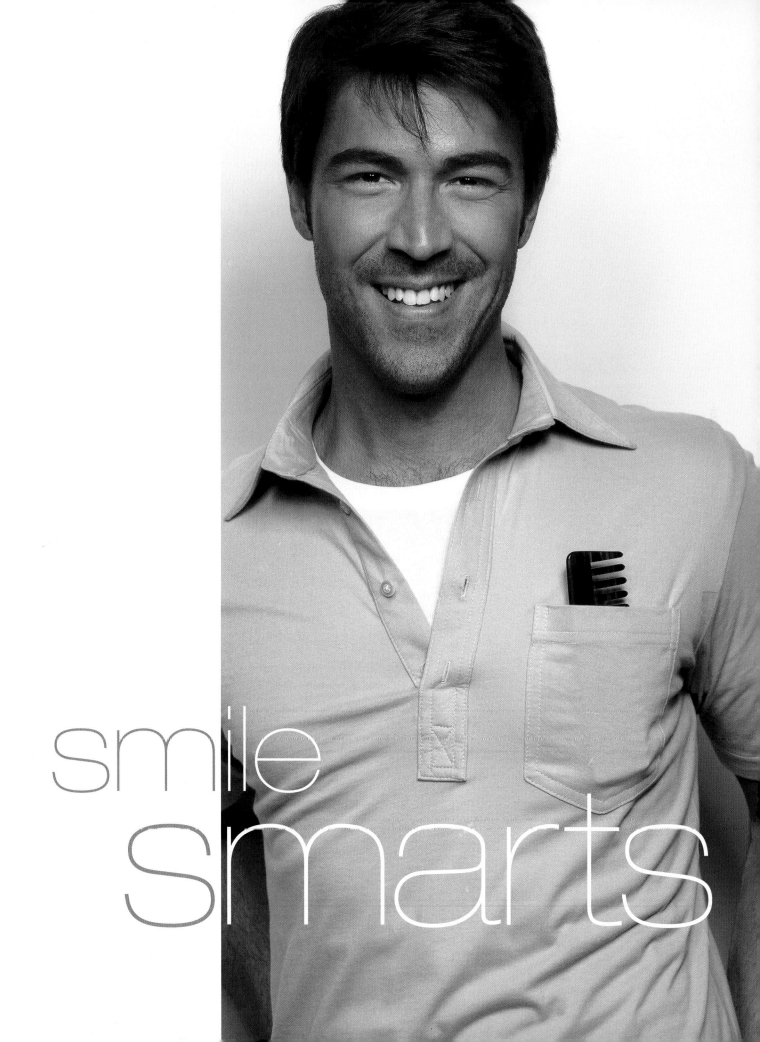

smile
smarts

Think braces are for kids? Well, it's never too late for a great smile. In fact, I wear them, but you'd never know it. Since I can't show up at work with a mouthful of metal, I decided to go with this new type of teeth straightening that involves a series of clear retainers you wear over the course of several months. I take them out when I'm on camera, eating, or brushing my teeth, but other than that, I wear them all day long and no one can tell. Of course, I've lost a few of these retainers in the past few months, which brings on a bit of déjà vu. Back in middle school, I lost my retainer and never told my parents, so my teeth shifted out of place. If I had only known then what I know now, I would have fessed up and had it replaced.

The simple truth about your teeth? Take care of them and they'll take care of you. I brush a few times a day, floss daily, and see my dentist on a regular basis. If I didn't, I'd be looking at a future of tooth decay, gum disease, and maybe even tooth loss. Not pretty.

Our society puts so much emphasis on straight, bright white teeth. Every celebrity has a perfect smile, but believe me, few are born that way. You don't need a movie star smile to be beautiful, although I know it's hard to feel your best if there's a problem with your teeth. Don't be afraid to visit a dentist and talk to him or her if you're feeling self-conscious. If you're embarrassed about the color of your teeth, discuss whitening, either in the dentist's office or using one of the many affordable at-home options. If your teeth need to be straightened, you have a lot of choices. Whatever the problem, your dentist is sure to have a solution.

Unfortunately, the worse your problem, the more expensive the solution. If you're afraid you can't afford the work, ask your dentist about a payment plan. You can also look in the phone book for a dental school in your area. Give them a call and see if they need patients. They may charge nothing, or just a nominal fee, if you volunteer to be worked on by a student.

kyanism

Nasty breath is rude. If someone's going to be in my face—in a good way (a makeup artist, facialist, or yoga teacher)—I always try to have a mint beforehand. But mints don't get to the root of the problem. Most people think bad breath comes from their stomachs, but often it's from the bacteria on their tongues. Every time you brush, remember to brush your tongue or use a tongue scraper. If that doesn't help, try a mint-flavored parsley oil capsule, available at most health food stores. You suck on it for a few minutes, then swallow. Parsley is a great breath-freshener.

teeth time with dr. salzer

I'm lucky to have a great dentist, Dr. Jennifer Salzer. I actually want to floss every day just to make her happy. She's got lots of no-nonsense advice about teeth, so I asked her to share her wisdom with you.

Kyan: Why should we visit our dentists every six months?

Dr. Salzer: At that point, even patients with excellent home care will have a certain amount of tartar and plaque they can't remove with brushing alone, so a good cleaning is necessary. Also, if there's any cavity formation, your dentist can take care of it before it becomes a problem.

Kyan: What constitutes good home care?

Dr. Salzer: The old standards—brushing and flossing.

Kyan: Any tips for better brushing?

Dr. Salzer: I like power toothbrushes because they really help the patients do more than they can do with a manual toothbrush. You also need to brush for two minutes to cleanse all the surfaces properly. Most people brush for only 20 seconds. I tell my patients to turn on some music and brush to a song. The average song is about two minutes.

Kyan: A lot of people hate to floss. What happens if you don't do it?

Dr. Salzer: Brushing doesn't remove the plaque between teeth and by the gum line. If you can incorporate flossing into your beauty regimen, it will become a routine and you'll do it automatically. Eventually, you'll feel weird if you don't floss. The real, scary result of neglecting to floss is tooth loss.

Kyan: Let's talk about whitening.

Dr. Salzer: The general rule is that your teeth should not be whiter than the whites of your eyes. Almost everyone can benefit to some degree from whitening because it will brighten your smile. That doesn't mean you have to do a full-on laser treatment; you can do something like whitening strips, which work really well.

Kyan: What about whitening toothpastes?

Dr. Salzer: They brighten teeth, but not by whitening. They contain agents that remove stains. They may not make a significant difference, but you can get a few shades lighter just by removing stains.

Kyan: What about more intensive things, like bleaching trays and lasers?

Dr. Salzer: These involve applying peroxide or bleach to lighten the actual color of the teeth. The results are amazing, especially when you do the laser treatment and the trays in combination. However, people need to realize that teeth whitening is not permanent. It needs to be touched up every six months, but you can do the touch-ups at home with whitening strips.

You can keep your teeth whiter by staying away from things that stain your teeth, like

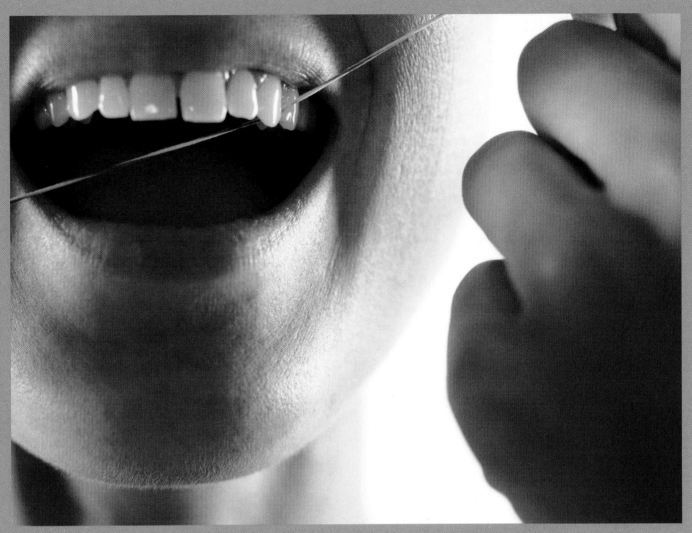

coffee, red wine, and tea. If you find that your teeth stain easily, but you want a glass of red wine, for example, try having a sip of water after every sip of wine.

Kyan: What are your options for straightening your teeth? You and I have talked about this a lot because you fitted me for my braces.

Dr. Salzer: There are traditional braces, clear braces, braces that go inside your teeth, and Invisalign, which is what you're doing. When teeth are crooked and misaligned, they look dirty and they're harder to clean. Straight teeth reflect light so beautifully.

Veneers are a quick fix and look great right away. Even though they can be beautiful, they're not natural, and everybody's really into natural beauty these days, especially you, Kyan. Sometimes, however, veneers are the only option if your teeth are not the right size or shape, or if you have tetracycline stains, which are permanent.

Kyan: Why is all this important?

Dr. Salzer: I'm a dentist, so of course I feel this way, but it's amazing how good a person can look when he or she has a nice smile. Of all the things that make a person beautiful—skin, hair, nails—your smile is number one.

lipstick tricks

Did you know that certain lipsticks make your teeth look whiter? Blue-reds and other blue-toned shades are best. Orange- and brown-toned colors make teeth look yellow.

feel-good flossing

If you really hate flossing, try one of those little wishbone-like devices that make it easier to floss. Don't cheap out when you buy your floss—a good brand makes all the difference. I love flat dental floss because it shreds less than old-fashioned floss, causes less gum bleeding, and won't hurt your finger as much.

afternoon delight

You should have a mini oral kit at your desk or in your bag containing toothpaste, toothbrush, floss, and alcohol-free mouthwash. Use it after lunch as a great way to freshen up and wake up.

toss it!

Take a good look at your toothbrush. Is it relatively new and clean with straight bristles? Or is it really gross with bristles that are splayed out and worn? I've invaded enough bathrooms to know that plenty of people use toothbrushes in their mouths that I wouldn't even use to clean my bathroom! If that's your case, buy a new brush, pronto. Buy several, in fact, so you have some on hand.

get whiter teeth

Laser teeth whitening takes place at a dentist's office or whitening center. Your lips are pushed away from your teeth with a plastic apparatus, then a bleach or peroxide solution is applied to your teeth. You put on protective goggles, then a laser is aimed at your teeth. It can be boring and uncomfortable, not because of the laser, but because of the position your mouth is in. Some dentists try to make the procedure entertaining by playing DVDs or providing video goggles. You'll be done before the flick is over.

The downside: the price.

Whitening trays are plastic pieces you fill with bleaching gel and fit over your teeth. If you get them from your dentist, they are customized for your mouth. Generally, you need to wear the trays for a minimum of four hours a day for however many days your dentist stipulates; some people opt to wear them while they sleep.

The downside: These can be a pain in the neck—and they can be a pain in the gums, as well. Laser whitening is much faster and efficient.

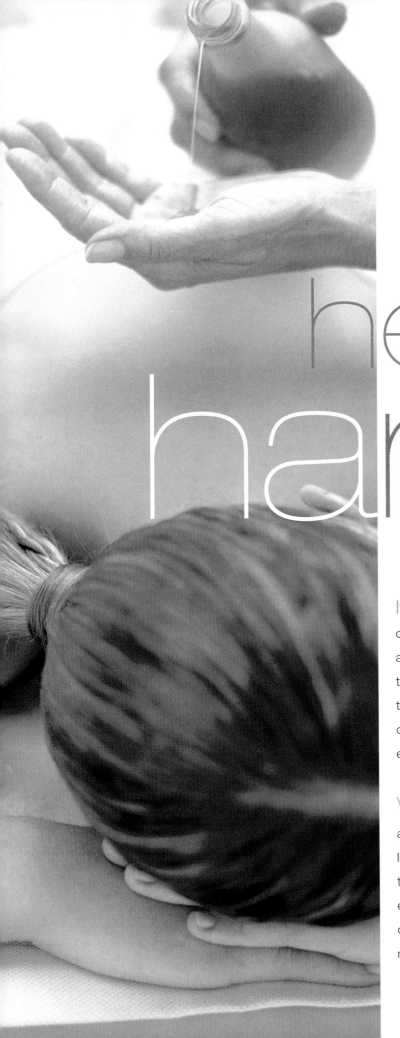

healing hands

If you've never had a massage, you don't know what you're missing. A lot of people are afraid to get one because it seems too intimate or they're wary of being touched by a stranger. While those fears are totally legitimate, they're worth overcoming. Massage is incredibly healing, both emotionally and physically.

where to begin

Do you want a nice, gentle massage that lets you forget about life for a while? Or something deeper and more therapeutic? These are two very different experiences and require a different set of skills on the part of the therapist, so it's good to identify what your needs and expectations are upfront.

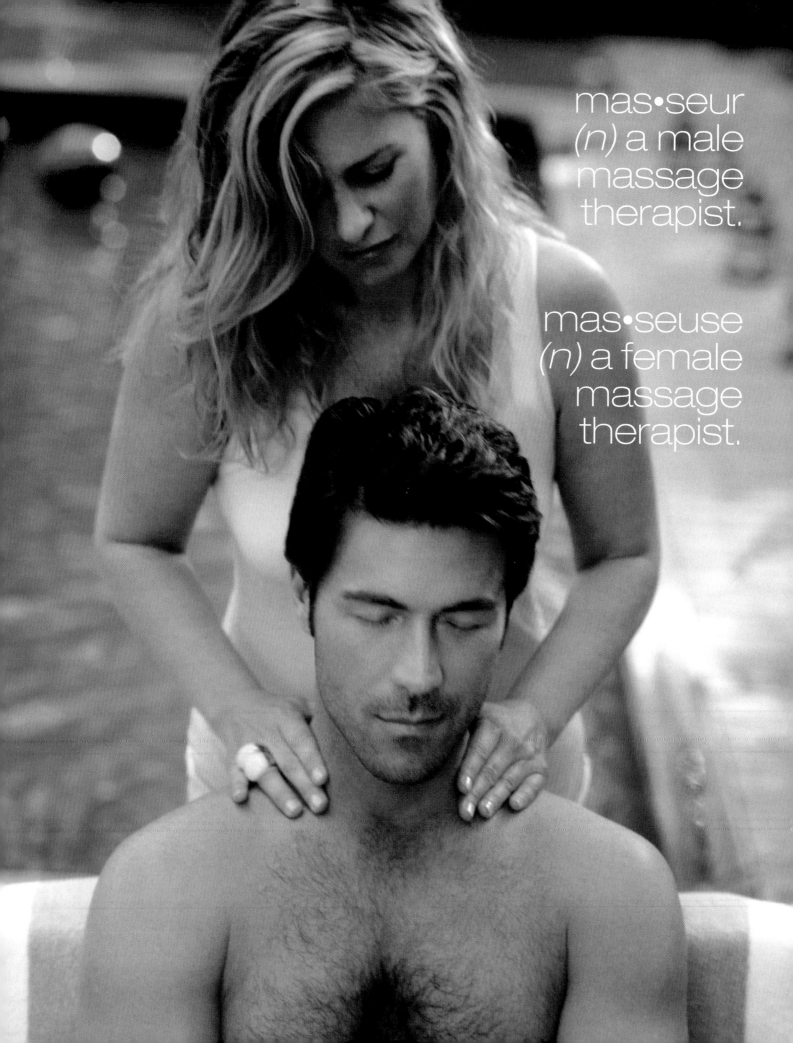

mas•seur
(n) a male
massage
therapist.

mas•seuse
(n) a female
massage
therapist.

When booking your massage, talk to the receptionist and ask for an explanation of the different massages available. There are extras that make one different from the next—intensity level, therapeutic value, length of time, or some type of accessory or product, such as hot stones or aromatherapy oils.

where can you find a good therapist? A recommendation from a friend or doctor is the best way to go. You can also look online or in the phone book for a local practitioner. If you need a therapeutic massage for serious muscular issues, you won't find what you're looking for at a spa or salon. Call a local chiropractor and ask for a recommendation. Be sure to explain that you want a "therapeutic" massage. Keep in mind that this type of work will be more painful than relaxing, but the benefits are worth it in the end.

massage 101

swedish massage The most basic massage, this serves as the foundation for most other types of massage. Great if you want to relax and get away from it all.

sports massage Also called neuromuscular therapy or deep-tissue massage, this is a very therapeutic method that involves a specific approach to each muscle. It's a great option if you have a minor injury, like a pulled muscle, or if your muscles are really tight. Since it's more invasive than Swedish massage, it can cause a bit of discomfort. After all, your therapist is literally ironing out your muscles. Remember to breathe through the pain.

hot stone massage To soothe your muscles and promote a positive energy flow, you are massaged with oil and warm, round stones. For further balance and relaxation, the stones are placed on your pressure points and chakra centers (we'll talk more about chakras on page 199). At some spas, cold or even frozen stones are incorporated as well.

aromatherapy massage This involves the use of scented oils to enhance your experience. Some fragrances, like peppermint, eucalyptus, and citrus, are stimulating; lavender is relaxing, and ylang-ylang and sandalwood are musky and sensual. Talk to your therapist about your scent likes and dislikes.

kyanism

Double the Pleasure During couples massage, you and your friend, boyfriend, or girlfriend get massaged side by side. You each get your own massage table and therapist. This is a great bonding experience, and it makes a wonderful gift idea (particularly for a friend who is interested in massage, but nervous about going alone).

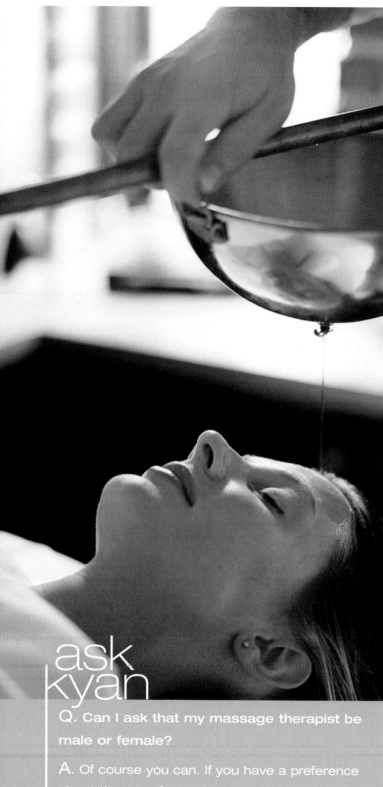

ayurvedic massage
This incorporates elements of Ayurveda (pronounced eye-yur-vay-da), which, simply put, is a health-care system for the mind, body, and spirit developed in India thousands of years ago. In Ayurveda, everything is composed of the five elements (space, air, water, fire, and earth), and those are manifested in human beings through one of three doshas—vata, pitta, or kapha. Most people correspond to one or sometimes two doshas, which are basically your body and personality types. Before an Ayurvedic treatment, your therapist may try to assess your dosha. Other terms you may hear include Abhyanga (a-bee-yan-ga), which is massage with warm oil to boost circulation and remove toxins, and Shirodhara (shir-o-dar-a), which involves pouring warm oil on your forehead (or your "third eye") to promote mental clarity and soothe the central nervous system.

reflexology
With this massage philosophy, specific points on your hands, feet, and ears refer to specific organ systems in your body. By massaging these points, you can alleviate pain or stimulate certain bodily functions.

the heat is on
If the spa has a sauna or steam room, use it before your massage so that you're loose and relaxed. Steam for a little bit, then shower. If you have sinus issues, the dry heat of the sauna is better. Time limit: 15 minutes. Take some cool water with you. If you feel light-headed or dizzy, get out. Make sure to wear flip-flops (yours or the ones provided) and bring an extra towel to sit on.

ask kyan

Q. Can I ask that my massage therapist be male or female?

A. Of course you can. If you have a preference about the sex of your therapist, that's totally fine. Just be sure to communicate this when you make your appointment. If you wait until you show up, the spa may not be able to accommodate your request.

good touch, bad touch

Most of your body will be covered with a large sheet or towel during your massage. The only exposed part is what the therapist is working on. It's important to establish boundaries. If you don't want the therapist touching a certain spot, simply say, "You know what? I don't like being touched there. Just right in here is great." If you feel the therapist is touching you in an inappropriate way, immediately tell him or her that you're uncomfortable.

You need to communicate what you want. Don't want to talk? Tell the therapist that you want to relax and drift away. Want the massage to be more intense, or less? Say so. Don't suffer in silence.

amateur hour

Massage can be a wonderful experience at home, too, whether you're giving or receiving. Dim lights, a few candles, and soothing music will set the mood. Have a friend, girlfriend, or boyfriend loosen up your tense shoulders, neck, and back. Even a fairly light touch can do the trick, so don't worry if you're lacking the strength or experience. Giving or receiving a massage means taking the time out of your day to pamper yourself or a friend, and that is never a bad thing.

the receiving end

As a student of massage, other therapists who worked the kinks out of me always said I was good at receiving massages. During the procedure, I always let go; I melted and focused on my breathing. There really is an art to enjoying massage. When you get a massage, try to let go and give in to the massage therapist's touch. You have to be in the moment; learn how to receive that touch and immerse yourself in it. Turn yourself over to the experience and you'll have an amazing experience.

clothes call

It's customary to get naked for your massage, but if you're modest, you should at least strip down to your panties. A bra will get in the way when the therapist works on your shoulders and back. Bottom line: Do what makes you comfortable.

ask kyan

Q. How can I tell if the pain I feel during a massage is good pain or bad pain?

A. Great question. With sports massage, therapeutic massage, or deep-tissue massage, discomfort is part of the deal. An even flow of breath can help. Breathe in and imagine your breath going to that spot, then breathe out and imagine the tension leaving with your breathe. Don't ever hold your breath.

how not to diet

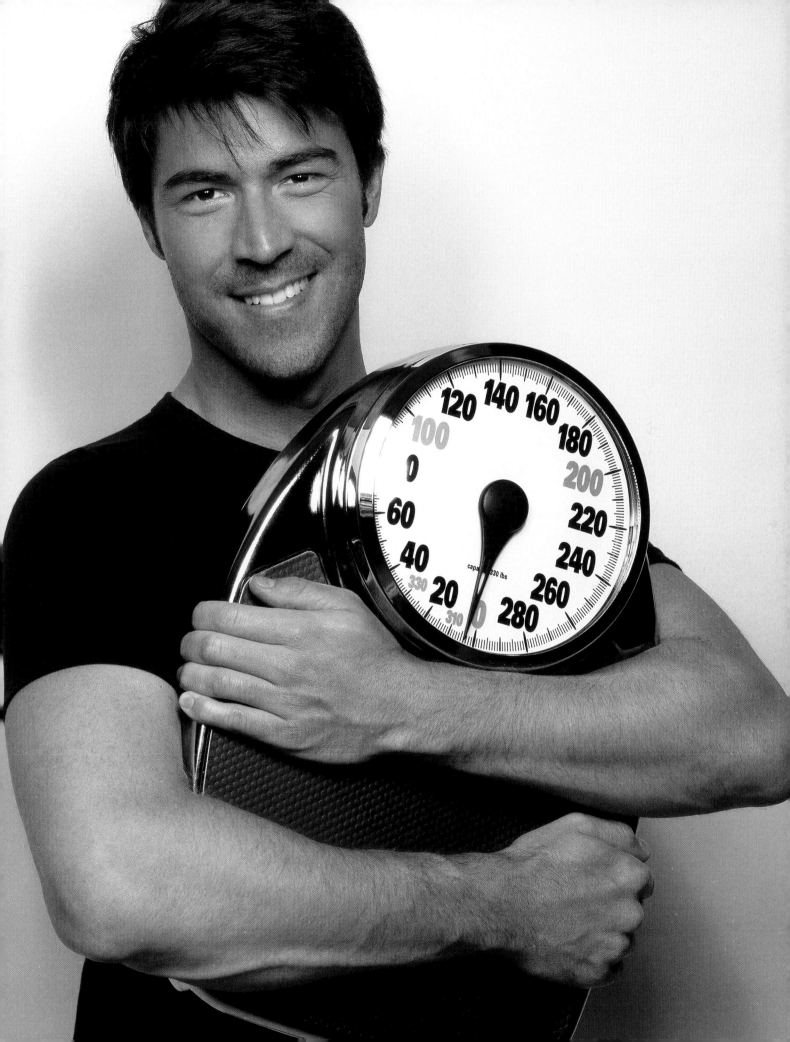

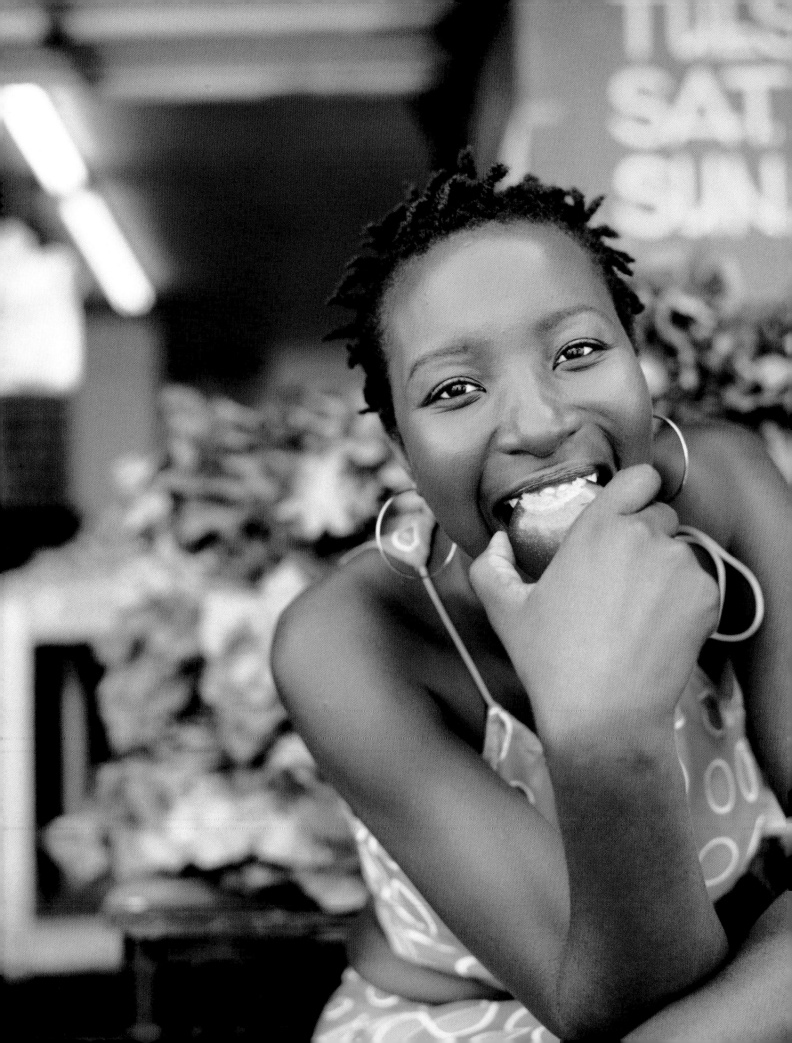

I certainly hope that the phrase "you are what you eat" is not true,

because I've been eating a little too much junk food lately. You know I hate excuses, but it's tough to keep to a healthy diet when you work long hours and you're stuck on a set. The food lady walks by with a tray of doughnuts and the next thing you know, you've had a doughnut for breakfast. When I'm eating the wrong foods, I feel sluggish and heavy—definitely low energy. When I eat right, it makes a huge difference in how I look and feel. So if my body and brain know this, why am I so tempted to reach for the bad stuff?

The reason is that you and I have an emotional connection to food. Sure, we eat to satisfy ourselves when we're hungry, but we also eat to deal with our stress, sadness, boredom, or anger. There's a chance you don't even know you're doing this.

I know, you probably think that you don't have time to plan your day around your meals. But that's not what I'm proposing. You shouldn't have to follow an extreme diet regimen amid all of your other responsibilities. I'm encouraging you to be conscientious of what you're eating, and realize that what you eat makes a huge impact on how you feel. Remember, beautified means that you feel good on the inside as well as on the outside. What better way of making sure of that than by fueling your body with the best possible foods? You deserve nothing less.

Eating right shouldn't have to be a struggle. In this chapter, I want to give you the tools to make smart food decisions, whether you're trying to loose weight, eat healthier, conquer your sweet tooth, or just feel better about yourself. At the same time, I want you to have a realistic relationship with food because it's such a great part of life. When you cook with your significant other, have dinner with your family, or meet your friends for drinks, you should be able to enjoy yourself, not stress over calories or carb content.

kyan's food rules

stop dieting! Successful eating is all about balance and moderation. Think in terms of long-term health and long-term results. Diets are temporary, which is why they so often fail. You need an everyday eating plan, not an "until I lose 10 pounds" plan.

start eating. Starving yourself won't get you anywhere. If you drastically cut back the amount of food you eat, you won't lose weight. Your body will go into starvation mode and hold on to every last pound. The fact is that eating on a regular basis helps your metabolism (the process by which your body breaks down food and burns up calories) stay elevated. Of course, you have to eat the right foods. Junk food and empty calories won't cut it.

breakfast is a must. Think about that first word—it means *break the fast.* By the time you wake up in the morning, you probably haven't eaten a thing in at least 10 hours. Just because you can last until lunch without food doesn't mean you should. Your body needs fuel! Set the tone for the day and jumpstart your metabolism by eating something healthy.

don't wait until you're hungry. If you're eating when you're hungry, you've waited too long. At that point, you're more likely just to grab whatever's in front of you. Your body instinctively wants something that will give it immediate energy—so you reach for that high-calorie blueberry muffin or greasy slice of pizza instead of something nutritious. On the flip side, don't eat so much that you become uncomfortably full.

eat whole foods. Fresh fruit and vegetables, grains, nuts, cheese, and other foods that aren't processed and full of refined sugar are the smart way to go.

three meals a day? forget it! That's the old rule. Five or six small meals throughout the day is a better idea. This way, your blood sugar never plummets, your metabolism is consistently elevated, and you don't need that quick snack fix. If it's hard to break the breakfast-lunch-dinner routine, try healthy snacks in between meals.

don't eat right before bedtime. Your digestion slows down after hours, especially when you sleep. Avoid late-night meals or snacking. If your schedule requires late nights, make sure you plan ahead.

pay attention. Read labels, and be aware of exactly what you're eating and *why* you're eating it. Make conscious food choices.

indulge from time to time. Depriving yourself of the food you want will make you cranky and eat more. But use common sense. There's a big difference between indulging in two cookies and overindulging in an entire box.

it's never too late to start. It doesn't matter what you weigh or how old you are. Make a change today and you'll be healthier tomorrow.

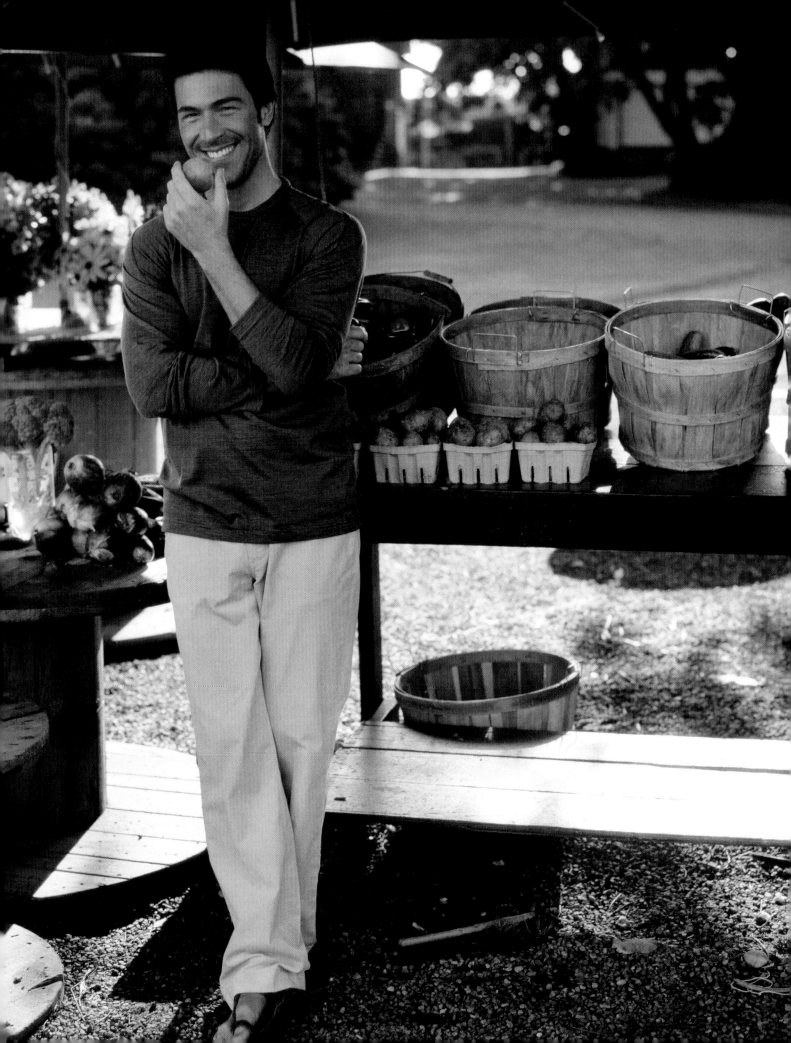

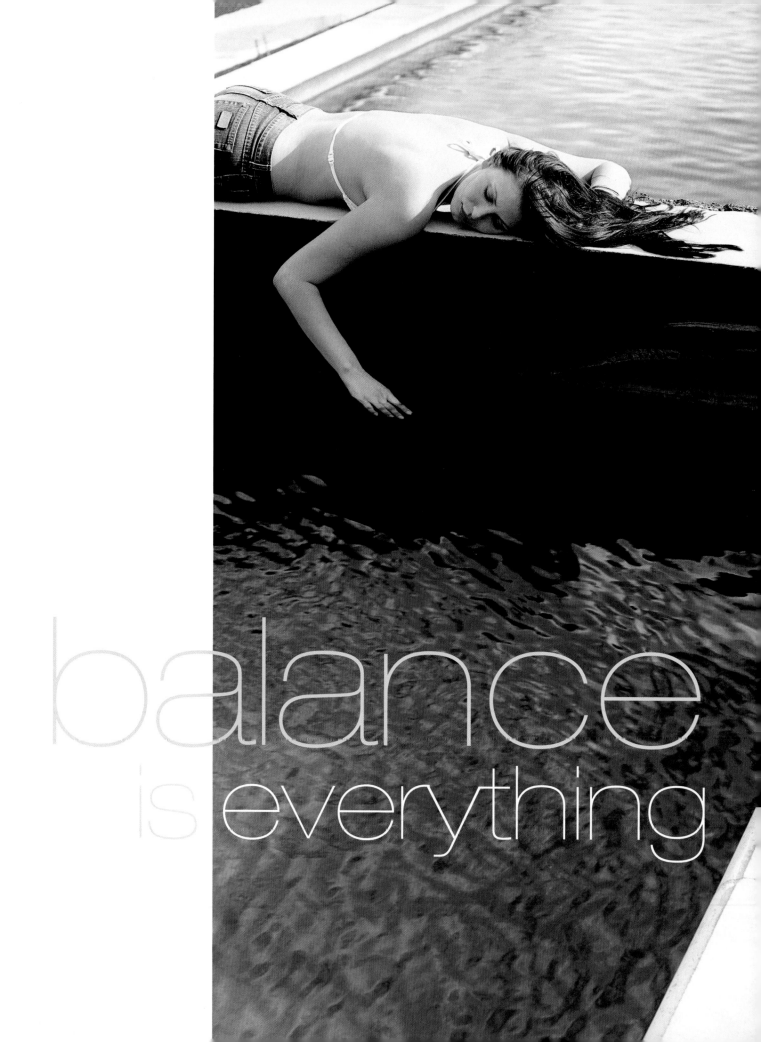

balance
is everything

I truly believe the secret to smart eating is balance, and by that, I mean five or six small meals a day that consist of equal parts lean protein (like chicken or fish), a complex carbohydrate (we'll explain just what that means later in the chapter), and vegetables. The meals are supplemented by healthy snacks of fruit, veggies, and/or nuts.

Here is an example of what I consider a perfect day's diet.

breakfast

- oatmeal (not instant)
- 2 scrambled egg whites with chopped scallions and smoked salmon

snack

- fresh fruit or unsalted seeds (I love pumpkin or sunflower)

lunch

- a baked turkey burger (mix in a ¼ cup of oatmeal before cooking)
- steamed broccoli or spinach drizzled with a teaspoon of olive oil
- small serving of brown rice

snack

- celery sticks with almond butter

dinner

- steamed or sautéed salmon fillet
- steamed green or yellow squash
- big green leafy salad with balsamic vinaigrette

set yourself up for success
No one sets out to fail, but it's amazing how we can sabotage ourselves. Take a look in your cabinets and in your fridge. I'm afraid to ask, but what kind of food is in there? Lots of junk food, soda, and processed stuff? Any fruits or vegetables?

know thyself.
If you struggle with willpower, don't bring tempting foods into the house. It's easier to put something back on the shelf at the supermarket than to exercise self-control in your kitchen in the middle of the night.

two rules about grocery shopping
Never shop while hungry. You'll end up buying more on impulse. If need be, don't walk down certain aisles. Skip the sections that make you go weak in the knees with temptation.

kyanism

Salad Sabotage
Don't ruin your salad by dumping high-fat, high-caloric dressing on top of it. The same goes for dips for your veggies or fruit. The dressings might be tasty, but they cancel out the benefits you're getting from the healthy stuff. A vinaigrette of balsamic vinegar and olive oil should be your first choice for salads. For a nutritious veggie dip, try hummus, a delicious purée of chickpeas, instead of fattening dairy-based dips.

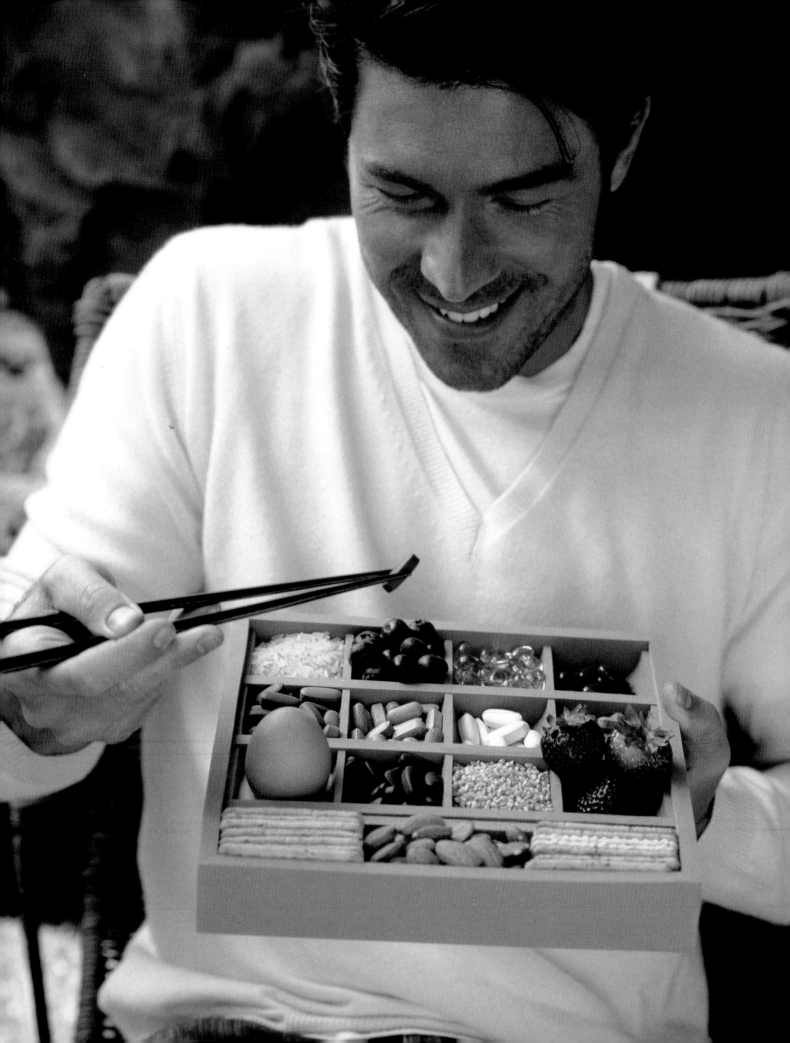

Never shop without a list. Once you're at the store, the list rules. Do not deviate from it. These are always the basics you'll always find on my grocery list:

Organic Turkish apricots • Strawberries • Bananas • Frozen mixed berries • Soy protein • Unsweetened soy milk • Unsweetened rice milk • Hummus • Almond butter • Celery • Broccoli • Spinach • Mixed greens • Raw, unsalted almonds • Pumpkin seeds • Salmon

Always have healthy options on hand—at home and at work—such as nuts, dried fruits, fresh fruit, and chopped-up vegetables. Maybe you buy fruit and veggies, but they go bad before you get around to eating them? Buy ready-to-eat fresh fruit salad, grapes, tiny carrots, sliced red peppers, pre-washed lettuce. You'll have less of an excuse because everything's right at your fingertips, ready to satisfy a food craving.

trendy diets

Is it me, or does it seem like everybody's following some hot diet or eating plan these days? Don't jump on a diet bandwagon. Trends are fine when it comes to clothes, movies, and music, but not your health. A diet needs to make sense for the long term and include lots of healthy foods. A diet that allows you to eat unlimited amounts of bacon but restricts fruits and vegetables can't be good. Although you might lose 10 pounds and fit into that new dress, dropping weight quickly is a surefire way to ensure that you'll have trouble keeping it off.

The popularity of these diets has made the issue of food so confusing. What can you eat? What can't you eat? So much of eating well comes down to common sense. Listen to your body and your brain.

good carbs, bad carbs

The word *carbohydrate* covers a lot of territory. A strawberry is a carb (although it's a healthy fruit first and foremost), but so is a slice of white sandwich bread that comes in a bag and stays fresh for three weeks because it's full of preservatives. Due to the popularity of certain anti-carb diets, all carbs mistakenly have been labeled as bad. How many people do you know who are "avoiding carbs"? Lots, I bet.

What you should avoid are simple or processed carbohydrates. These are sugary and/or starchy foods that your body breaks down quickly for instant energy. They cause your blood sugar to spike quickly, then come crashing down—bringing you down with it, not to mention your metabolism. Of course, simple carbohydrates are the foods we crave, stuff like cookies, brownies, breads, muffins, pasta, and soda. High taste factor, but not much nutritional value. Some of these are even empty calories, meaning they'll make you feel full, but they won't provide your body with any nutrition.

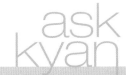

ask kyan

Q. Are organic foods better for you than nonorganic?

A. Despite what some food manufacturers claim, organic is better. For a product to be labeled organic, it must be raised, grown, or produced in a way that limits the use of pesticides, chemicals, and drugs. I'll take a grain-fed chicken over a caged-up bird pumped full of hormones and antibiotics any day. Same goes for fruits and vegetables that aren't sprayed with pesticides or altered genetically. Any time you can purchase or consume organic food, go for it.

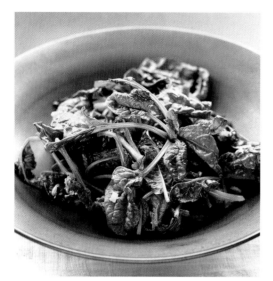

The good carbs are known as complex carbohydrates and include fruits, vegetables, grains, and beans. (Beans are a source of protein, too, so they're an essential component to a healthy diet.) Good carbs also get broken down by the body to provide energy, but the process takes much longer compared to simple carbs. As a result, you get the energy you need without the dramatic highs and lows. Plus, complex carbs are rich in fiber, which helps make you feel fuller faster and prevents your body from converting too many calories into fat.

fruits and veggies

I don't know about you, but these were not a big part of my diet as a child. I was a picky eater who pretty much existed on Spaghetti-O's, grilled cheese sandwiches, and all sorts of sugary cereals. I didn't like vegetables at all. My poor mother, in a valiant attempt to get me to eat something healthy, would cut up yellow squash, put it in my mashed potatoes, and tell me it was butter. I fell for it every time, until I got old enough to know better.

Today, I try to eat at least three servings of fruit and vegetables each day, but I know it's not easy for everyone to do so. Maybe you weren't raised to eat that way, you don't like fruits and vegetables, or you're always eating on the go. If you fit into one of these categories, try the tip I mentioned earlier about having cut-up, ready-to-eat fruits and veggies on hand. Or try sneaking them into your diet like my mom did. Ask for some broccoli or peppers on your pizza, throw some fruit into your smoothie, or get some lettuce or tomato on your sandwich at lunch. Anything is better than nothing.

no grain, no gain

Grains have certainly gotten a bad rap as part of this whole anti-carb movement, which is really unfortunate. They're delicious and a great source of fiber and certain vitamins and minerals. Because many of us didn't grow up eating grains, we tend not to eat a lot of them, or eat the wrong ones. Many of us choose white rice, which starts out in life as a good grain, but is stripped of all its nutrients. Brown or wild rice is a much better choice. Other good grains? Quinoa (pronounced keen-wah) sounds exotic but is tasty and easy to make. Bulgur, which is found in tabbouleh, a delicious Middle Eastern dish, and oatmeal (but not the instant kind) are good, too. Anything billed as a "whole grain" is great.

protein power

Carbs, as we discussed, are burned up quickly by your body; protein takes longer for the body to digest and provides a steady supply of energy. A lot of women I know are totally focused on eating lots of protein. Egg whites for breakfast, chicken breast for lunch, fish for dinner. Lean proteins are great for you, but don't focus on them to the exclusion of other important food groups. Too much protein can be bad for your kidneys and liver. You need a mix of complex carbohydrates and lean protein to keep your body energized.

too skinny?

It's hard to believe, but there are people who have trouble gaining weight. It's easy to consider them lucky, but really thin people don't see it that way. They're as self-conscious as those who are overweight. If you want to put on a few pounds, you need to consume extra calories. Just make sure these are healthy calories, not empty ones, and exercise with weights, so the pounds are distributed evenly.

dairy queen

That certainly doesn't describe me. I'm a bit lactose intolerant, so I tend to avoid dairy products. Instead of regular milk, I use soy milk in my coffee and smoothies. All soy milks are not created equal, so read the ingredient label when grocery shopping. Some of them taste good because they're sweetened with brown rice syrup, which is a type of sugar. Buy the unsweetened kind instead.

If you like regular milk, make sure you're not drinking whole milk, which has way too much fat. A much better choice is low-fat or skim milk.

If you're drinking milk for the calcium, there are other calcium sources that deliver even more of the essential mineral, like spinach, kale, and other dark, leafy green veggies.

fat versus fiction

We've been programmed to believe that all fats are bad. Some are truly bad for you, like the saturated fats you find in red meat, butter, and whole milk, and trans-fats, which are created through a chemical process. Trans-fats are found in margarine, certain baked goods, potato chips, and vegetable shortening. These can lead to clogged arteries and high blood pressure. But some fats are good, specifically unsaturated fats. These are necessary for healthy skin, hair, and nails, as well as the absorption of certain vitamins. Sources of unsaturated fats include olive oil, almonds, avocados, salmon, fish oil, and flaxseed oil.

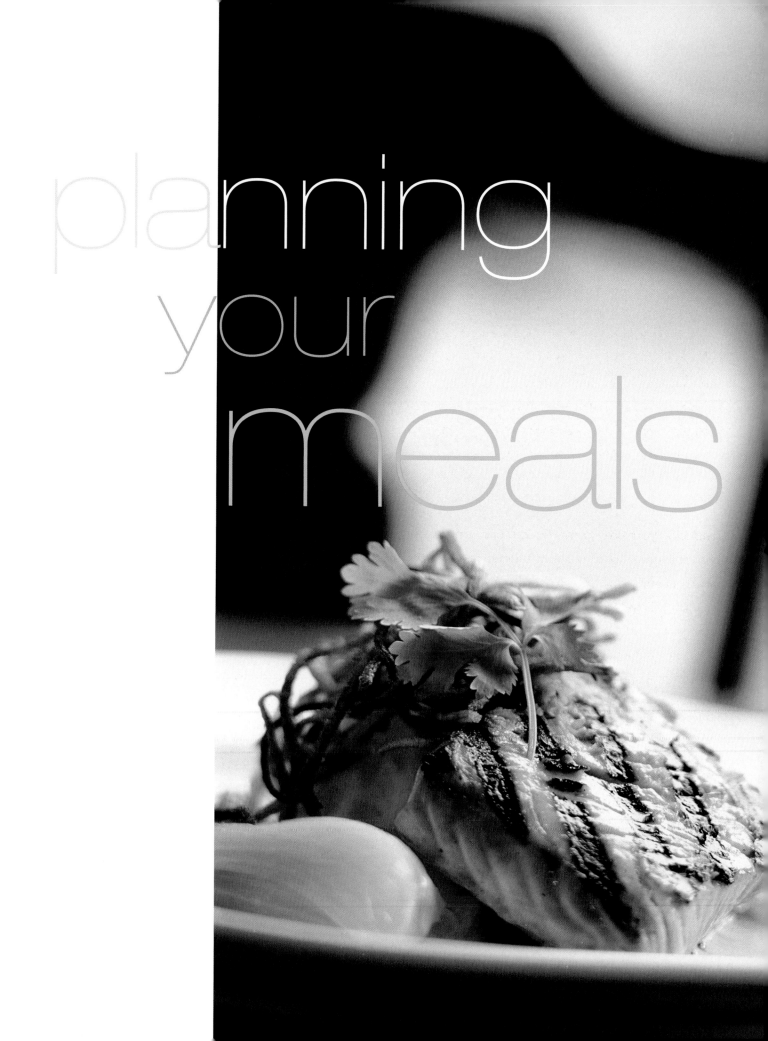

planning your meals

Remember when I talked earlier about setting yourself up for success? When it comes to your diet, the less you leave to chance, the better. Unless you travel a lot, you probably have a pretty set routine. On Sunday night, plan what you're going to eat for the next seven days. Think about the different places where you shop and eat and write down the healthiest options at each. Plan your snacks and beverages as well.

When you go out to eat, don't read the entire menu. Quickly scan it until you find something healthy, then stop reading. You'll be less tempted to order something naughty. If you're dining with like-minded people, ask to have the bread basket taken away. Or take one piece, *then* ask for it to be taken away. When the waiter or waitress brings the dessert menu, don't even look at it. If your fellow diners order dessert and you can't bear to sit there and watch them eat, see if someone will split dessert with you. Or better yet, order a bowl of plain berries. No cream on top! Sorbets can be a healthy choice, as long as they're made from puréed fruit, not sugar, flavoring, and coloring.

The idea isn't to deprive yourself, but to make better choices.

counting calories

The classic way to lose weight is by reducing your caloric intake. Lots of people have had success this way, and if you're looking to drop a few pounds, maybe this is the option for you. But how many calories should you consume each day? I've heard different advice from different dieticians. Some recommend that the average woman consume no more than 1,400 calories daily, others recommend between 1,600 and 2,200. Not only is this confusing; it doesn't specify what's right for an individual's body type, activity level, or metabolism. Some people are lucky to have a fast metabolism; others were born with a slow one. If you've ever wondered why certain people can eat lots of food and never gain a pound, while others seem to gain weight just by looking at food, it has to do with their metabolism. Protein consumption speeds up your metabolism, as does exercise; sugar, lack of sleep, and even aging can slow it down.

The bottom line on calories: Do what feels right for you. If you need to lose weight, you should consume less and work out more.

Taking the time to really enjoy food is a luxury some of us don't have. Maybe you're too busy trying to get out the door or you're trying to feed your kids and yourself at the same time. I totally understand that. But make an effort to focus on your food and not multitask while you eat. Take a bite and then put

kyanism

Water Works Aside from the wonderful hydrating effects that water has on your skin, it also can play a powerful role in terms of your appetite and food consumption. Drink water throughout the day and have a small glass 15 minutes before a meal. It will make you feel more full, so you'll consume less food. And, no, soda and juice are not adequate substitutes for H_2O.

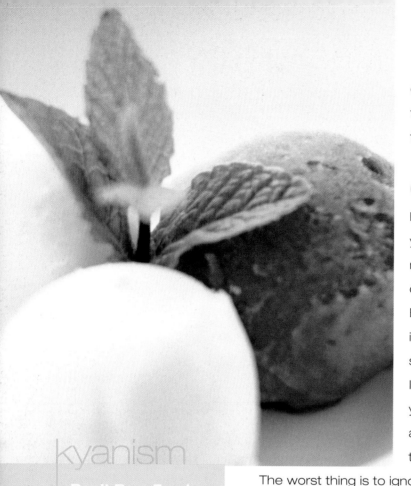

down your utensils. Chew slowly and think about the flavors you're experiencing. You'll become fuller faster and you'll probably eat less.

constant cravings

I've heard that cravings disappear after 10 minutes if you don't give in to them. Whoever said this must not crave much. I've had cravings that I can't get out of my head for days. The key is not to give in. Easier said than done, I know. You want that pint of ice cream? Don't go to the store and buy it. Find something distracting to do, like painting your nails. It takes a while for all 10 fingers to dry, so that limits your activity. Same with deep-conditioning your hair and putting on a face mask. You won't be tempted to run to the corner store looking like that.

The worst thing is to ignore your cravings and then totally fall off the wagon by bingeing on the object of your obsession. It's better to have a few bites than the entire thing—just make sure you have the willpower to stop after the second or third bite.

clean your plate

It's a sin to waste food. If you had a mother like mine, you've heard that expression so much, it's ingrained in your psyche. I'm sure we all agree with the sentiment, especially in a world where people go hungry. But cleaning your plate out of guilt is a bad idea that inevitably results in overeating. As a solution, take smaller portions, wrap up leftovers, and when you eat out, ask for a doggy bag. Pay attention to how you feel and simply stop eating when you are reasonably full.

sweet tooth

When you eat a lot of sweets, it's easy to get into the cycle of overeating. Your blood sugar spikes then plummets, so you need something to get it up again and you just keep eating. Once you start this cycle, it's difficult to stop. The way I deal with my sweet tooth is to eat small meals throughout the day to avoid ever getting really hungry, so I don't look to junk food for a quick fix. It's not a crime to have a piece of chocolate or a bite of cake. Just know when enough is enough and don't rely on sweets to make you feel satisfied. Learn the art of moderation!

kyanism

Don't Be a Food Bore Nothing's more tiresome than someone who's always on a diet *and* always talking about what or where they cannot eat. Don't let your diet dictate your social life. If you're meeting friends for dinner and drinks and you know the meal choices are pretty unhealthy, eat a salad or a healthy snack before heading out, and then order a soup or an appetizer. Don't make a big deal out of your dietary decisions —and don't make your friends feel bad if they're making different decisions now.

smart substitutions

Avoid products labeled low-fat, no-fat, fat-free, light, or "lite." (The only exception to this rule is dairy products; "whole" dairy products do have too much fat.) A lot of these foods are packed with sugar and chemicals to improve the taste, and they're not necessarily lower in calories—just lower in fat. You're better off having a bite or two of the food that contains fat than "fake food" loaded with substantial amounts of sugar and chemicals.

Here are some substitutions you can try. Some of the alternatives offer lower-fat and lower-calorie options, and others offer higher nutritional value and lower amounts of processed sugar.

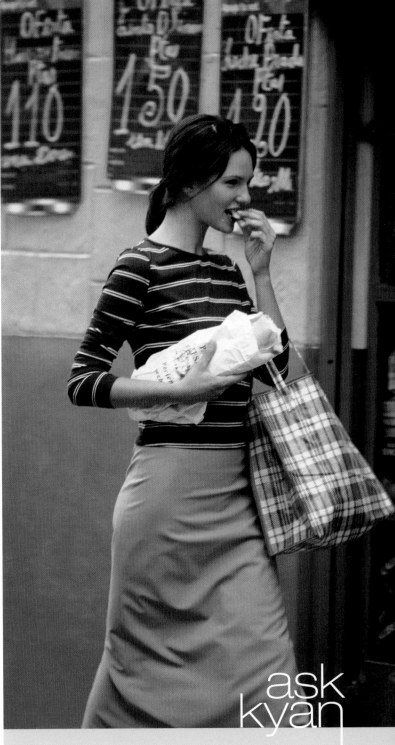

IF YOU LIKE:	TRY:
Soda	Fruit-flavored seltzer
Pretzels	Oat-bran pretzels
White bread	Whole-grain wheat bread
Ice cream	Fresh fruit sorbet
Bacon	Turkey bacon
Instant oatmeal	Irish oatmeal
Buttered popcorn	Plain popcorn
Flavored yogurt	Plain, low-fat yogurt with fresh, diced fruit
Chocolate bar	A few squares of dark chocolate
Pasta	Whole-wheat pasta
Candy	Dried organic apricots (sugarless)
Salted peanuts	Raw unsalted almonds

ask kyan

Q. Sometimes I experience an energy slump in the middle of the day, and I'm tempted to get candy or some other snack from the vending machine. What can I do to avoid this?
A. Unfortunately, vending machines tend to be stocked with foods that are high in sugar and fat and low in nutritional value. Fight the urge by keeping your own supply of nuts and dried and fresh fruits nearby. A banana is a great solution if you're feeling hungry and low-energy.

vitamins: a to z

I'm a big believer in taking vitamins. Most people don't eat enough fruits and vegetables, and even if they do, they may not be getting all the nutrients they should.

Every day, you should take a multivitamin that provides 50 to 100 percent of the daily value of key nutrients. I prefer shopping for vitamins at the health food store because they always have a good selection. Make sure to read the label and see if it includes essentials such as folic acid, calcium, iron, selenium, zinc, and vitamins A, B6, B12, C, and E. Look for vitamins that are free of artificial colors and flavors, sugar, preservatives, and sodium. You don't need junk like that in your vitamins. You also can take additional supplements. A calcium supplement, for example, is a great idea if osteoporosis runs in your family. Or take a vitamin C supplement if you're prone to colds. Read the label to see if you should take the vitamin or supplement with a meal or on an empty stomach.

on the go

A fast-food meal of a burger, fries, and soda is so calorie-laden it can surpass your entire suggested daily caloric intake. Today, fast-food chains are making an effort to offer healthy meals. If your only option is to eat at one of these places, order a salad, grilled chicken, and a bottled water.

French fries and onion rings, by the way, are not vegetables—they're devoid of nutrition and loaded with trans-fats.

serving size

Chances are you eat a lot more food than your body requires. The average restaurant meal could feed you for an entire day. In general, a serving size is equivalent to a deck of cards. I've seen steaks meant for one person that could easily feed a family of four. Even the average bagel is way oversized.

If you get smart about portion control, you won't have to deprive yourself of certain foods. Just because a store or restaurant has decided what the portion size is doesn't mean you need to eat the entire thing. When you go to the movies, avoid the "value" deals. Getting the large popcorn and the large soda might seem like a bargain, but it will cost you in the long run.

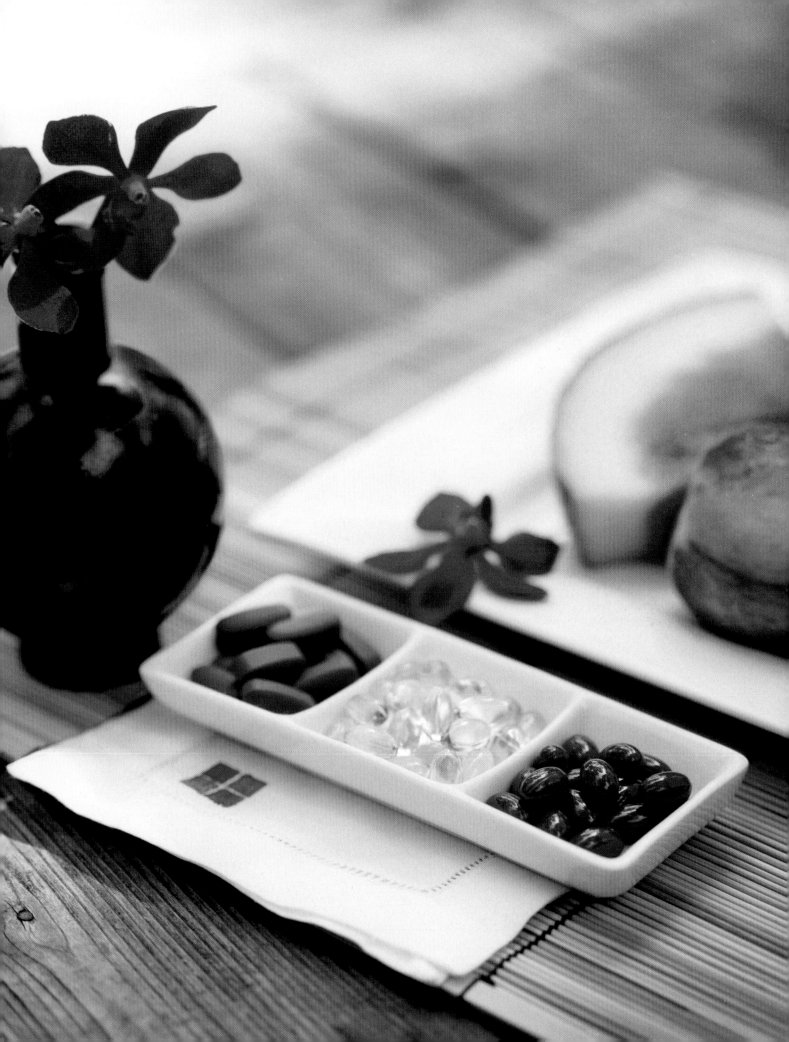

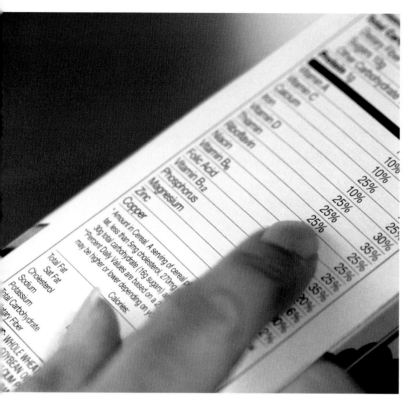

reading labels

Do you read the label of every food you buy? If you don't, you should. It's a great habit to get into because you'll really understand what you're putting in your body. It's amazing what certain foods contain and we don't even know it.

In general, the shorter the ingredients list, the better. It means the food is less processed and contains fewer chemicals and preservatives. Contents are listed in descending order, so the first ingredient is key. If sugar is the first ingredient, the food contains more sugar than anything else.

When it comes to breads, look for the words *whole-wheat flour.* An ingredient that reads *wheat flour* is 25 percent whole-wheat and 75 percent white flour (which has been stripped of any nutrients).

Pay particular attention to the serving size on the label. The calories and other nutritional information refer to one serving, and you'll be surprised how many servings are in certain packaged foods. One pint of ice cream can contain four servings. Certain candy bars contain two servings. If you eat the entire thing, you need to multiply everything by the serving size. Three servings, 200 calories per serving? That's 600 calories total.

The "calories from fat" category is also important because your daily diet should not consist of more than 30 percent fat. That's the current recommended number, but I think it's too high. Aim for 25 percent or lower. As I mentioned, look out for saturated and trans-fats, both of which are bad fats. Food manufacturers aren't required to list trans-fats yet, so you might not find these on the label even if the food contains them. Basically, you'll have to judge based on the ingredients and overall fat content.

ask kyan

Q. What is food combining?

A. This is a practice in which certain foods are eaten at different times because they are digested at different rates. People who practice this believe that it causes more successful digestion because it allows the body to process nutrients at their fullest extent, and it prevents indigestion. This is just one example, but someone practicing food combining would never eat fruit, which is digested quickly, with protein, which takes longer to process. They believe combining the two would delay the digestion of the fruit and cause it to ferment. This practice is mostly followed by vegans and vegetarians. Some nutritionists scoff at the concept, and others recommend it. If this sounds like something that makes sense for your diet, you should investigate further.

sugar baby

Once you start reading labels, you'll be shocked to find out how much sugar is in the food you eat every day. There's sugar in certain wheat breads, soups, deli meats, and other items you'd never expect to contain sugar. Another problem is that sugar rarely appears on the ingredients list as sugar. Instead, it's called sucrose, dextrose, fructose, maltose, cane sugar, corn syrup, or dozens of other names. Would you recognize polysaccharide as a sugar? Or sorghum? Most people wouldn't. That's why it's important to look at the entire label. If you can't find sugar on the ingredients list, check to see if it is listed under the total carbohydrates category.

As I mentioned earlier, sugar represents nothing but useless, empty calories that cause your blood sugar to spike and send your cravings into overdrive. Sugar also robs your body of nutrients because certain vitamins and minerals are needed to process it.

A number of prominent dermatologists believe that sugar is bad for your skin and speeds the aging process. I know it's almost impossible to cut sugar from your diet entirely, so here's a goal: Don't eat anything sugary during your final meal of the day. This means forgoing dessert and alcohol with dinner. Don't worry, you can have these treats during the day, if you must. You should go to bed with something healthy in your belly, like protein or complex carbs.

veggies rule

A few years ago, when I was studying massage and getting serious about my spiritual journey, I became a vegan. A vegan diet consists of foods solely from the plant world, so not only is meat avoided, but so are eggs and dairy. I found that I didn't have enough energy on the vegan diet, so I stopped eating that way after a year. Looking back, I think I was really enthusiastic about the concept, but I didn't really understand how to live that way.

Being a vegan or a vegetarian is a major commitment that requires you to do your homework and plan your meals. It's easier to be a vegetarian these days; even fast-food restaurants offer salads and veggie burgers. It's much harder to be a vegan. You don't eat out as much, unless you're dining with other vegan friends, and you wind up preparing a lot of your own food. I'm not saying this to discourage anyone. Both veganism and vegetarianism can be meaningful ways of life. The amount of resources in terms of food, water, and land devoted to raising livestock is pretty shocking, so an animal-free diet means you're really giving back to the planet.

the diet health connection

My nutrition guru is Dr. Steven Margolin, a chiropractor and wellness expert. He really practices what he preaches. That's just an expression, though—he never preaches; he's more into making suggestions. Like most of us, Dr. Margolin wasn't born into a family of nutritious eaters. His childhood was filled with Pop-Tarts, peanut butter and jelly on white bread, soda, candy bars, pizza, and pasta. He suffered terribly as a kid from allergies during pollen season, and he always had a runny nose and was always getting sick. As he got older, he started eating better, but he always had low energy. Years later, when he was a practicing chiropractor, he attended a nutrition seminar that changed his life and, subsequently, the lives of several patients.

The seminar covered the various toxins in the foods we eat, and it included detailed instructions on how to detox. He went on a strict detox diet and saw some major changes: He lost 25 pounds, his skin glowed, he had more energy than ever, and most important, his allergies went away.

He's put me on a version of his detox diet in order to get my eating back on track. (Remember when I told you at the beginning of this chapter that I've been eating too much junk lately?) Honestly, keeping to the diet was really hard at first. I had to give up a lot of things that I love: coffee and wine were the hardest. I also love sugar and carbs, and they're out of the question because they trigger cravings. The whole idea behind detox is balancing your energy and blood sugar levels. After just a few days on Dr. Margolin's detox diet, I felt better. My skin looked better, despite the fact that I was working long days, and I had more energy. If you can stick to a diet like this, you'll notice that your cravings become less severe and you're not dying for sweets and snacks.

Detoxing is normally an extreme process. Consult with your doctor or nutritionist before starting a detox regimen.

ask the doctor

Dr. Margolin's detox diet is fairly involved, but there are some easy-to-follow elements of it that everyone can benefit from. I sat down with Dr. Margolin and asked if he would share his advice and wisdom to help you eat better *and* feel better.

Kyan: If someone wants to make a change in their diet, where do they start?

Dr. Margolin: I ask three main questions. Is this person making conscious choices to bring nutritious food into their system? Is this person making the choices, whether conscious or not, to bring lots of toxins into their body? Then, is their current diet and eating regimen going to support them in feeling 100 percent? The most important step is changing the way you think. Because of my detoxing experiences, I've changed the way I look at certain foods. I no longer crave the same foods I did as a child. This takes a lot of mind control, but the results are extraordinary.

Kyan: So what's the first step?

Dr. Margolin: The first thing everyone can do is think about the liquids that go into their bodies. That means drinking more water and more clean beverages. A clean beverage would be a pure fruit juice that hasn't been sweetened, although it can be diluted with water. Look at the label. Labels are there for a reason. Then decrease the amount of coffee, alcohol, and soda that you drink. These are what I call "unserving" beverages because they are not going to serve your body in functioning better; rather they're going to create a chemical change in your body through the sugar, the caffeine, and all the artificial flavoring and coloring.

Kyan: What's next?

Dr. Margolin: Then I bring to people's attention the three categories of food they should start to decrease or eliminate from their diet. The first is fried foods. When you heat an oil to fry food, it becomes rancid and your body doesn't know how to get rid of it. Second category: sugar. Refined sugar is a drug. People get addicted to it. Again, start reading labels to see what your foods really contain and look for foods that are naturally sweetened.

Kyan: What are some acceptable sweeteners?

Dr. Margolin: Evaporated cane juice is probably the most common natural sweetener. Other types include maple syrup, stevia, barley malt, and turbinado, the sugar that comes in those little brown packs. It's not as concentrated as white refined sugar. There are plenty of naturally sweetened foods on the market.

Kyan: What's the final category to avoid?

Dr. Margolin: Highly processed foods—things like breads and desserts. If it comes in a box or a bag or a can, read the label. See how many ingredients are in it. If it contains a ton of seemingly meaningless things (items you've never heard of and can barely pronounce), it probably contains a lot of preservatives and additives, which makes it highly processed. Your body's going to have a difficult time breaking all of that down and it will have to work a lot harder to process it. Eating more fresh food will make a difference.

Kyan: All of those steps will improve how someone feels?

Dr. Margolin: Absolutely. If you were to take care about the beverages you drink and be aware of decreasing or eliminating those two categories of food we just talked about, you'll experience a huge shift in the way you feel. Your energy will change, and your metabolism will change.

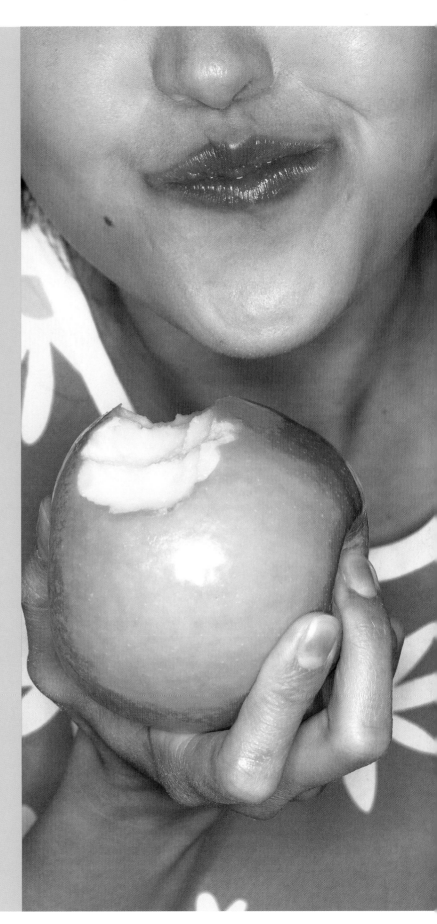

shape
it
up

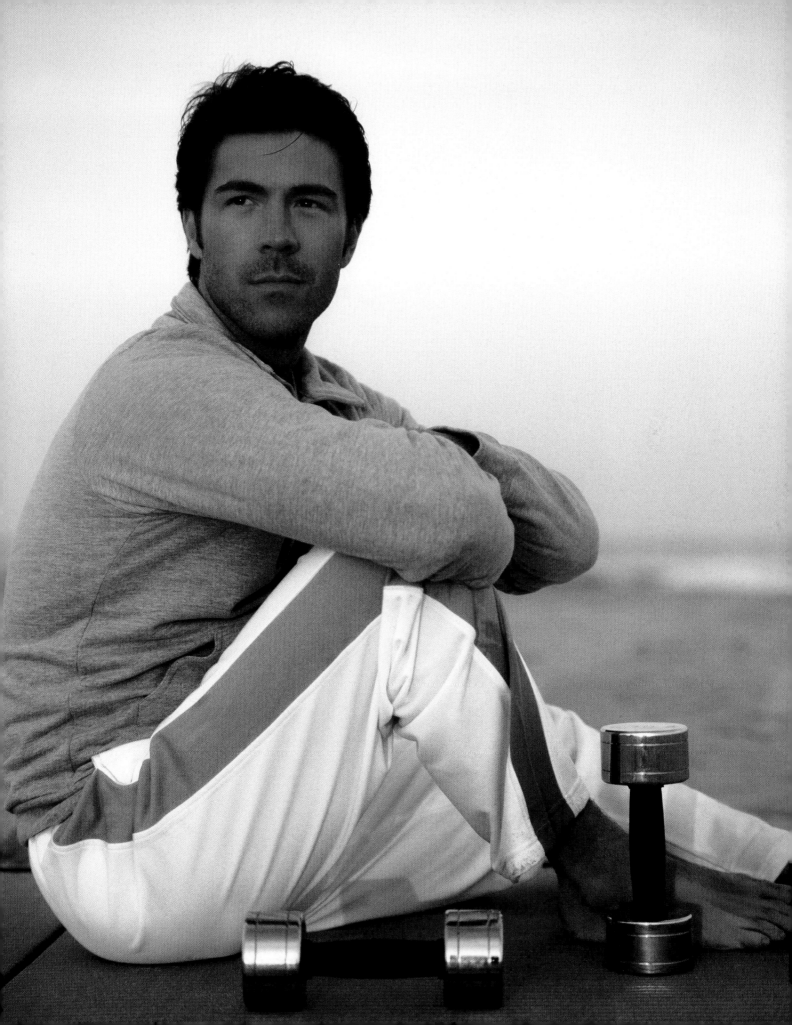

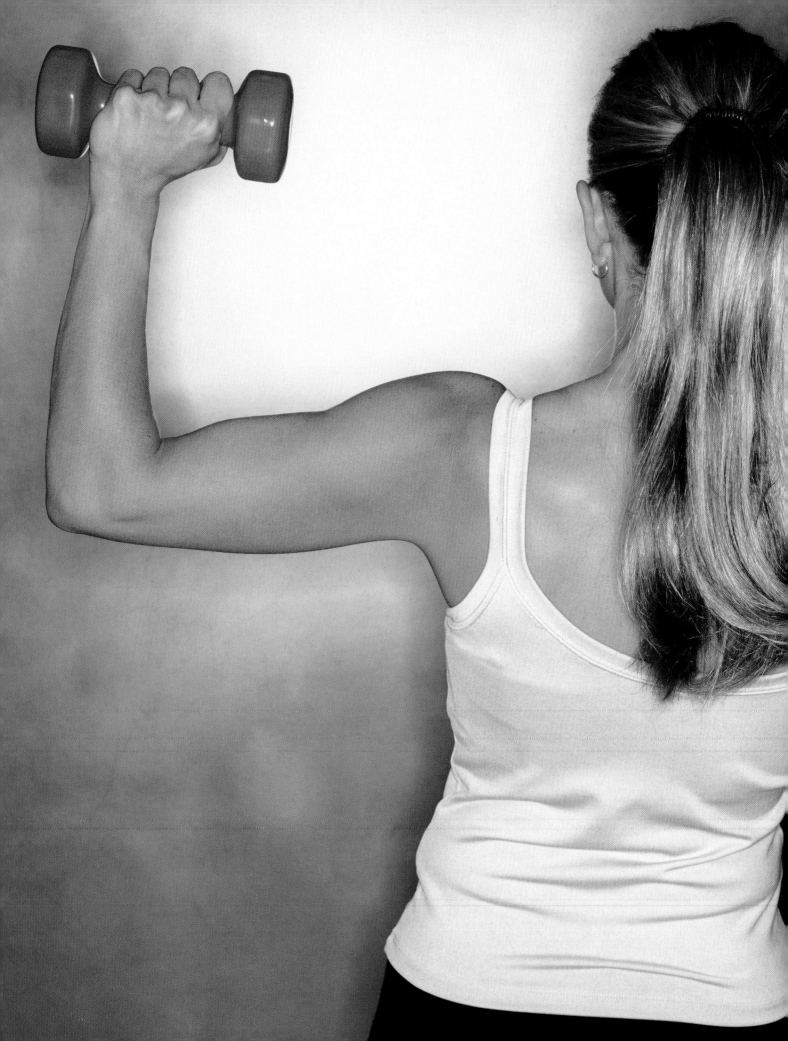

I know this won't come as a surprise, but growing up, I was not a jock.

I wasn't athletic at all—no basketball, baseball, track, or soccer. Then somewhere around the age of 16, I decided I was tired of being skinny and awkward. I knew intuitively that I'd feel better about myself if I did something with my body, so I got a cheap weight bench plus some barbells and dumbbells and started working out in the garage with a friend of mine. I followed the advice in fitness magazines, and pretty soon I noticed a difference.

I've tried to be consistent about working out ever since, although I've certainly gone through periods where I didn't exercise at all. Now that my schedule is so crazy, I'll admit that *work* makes it difficult to *work out*. But I know myself and I know my body—I feel better and I look better when I find the time.

Today, when people talk about their bodies, they're mainly focused on diet, but I don't believe you can separate diet and exercise. You're much better off focusing on fitness before you change your eating habits, because it's much easier to start a workout routine than a diet. Why? Because once you get moving, endorphins are released, which help you feel good, and you have more energy. You'll also find that you crave different foods as you get more fit. After you walk, do some in-line skating, or take a yoga class, you don't want a pint of ice cream or a can of diet soda. You want a salad, fruit, or something healthy.

Being fit is an essential component of being beautified. Seeing muscle tone, being able to walk up a few flights of stairs without losing your breath, and knowing that you're choosing outfits to complement rather than hide certain areas of your body are incredibly empowering. It makes you confident to know that you're pushing your body to look its best, and as you get more fit, your confidence will build. Yes, working out can be time-consuming and inconvenient. But many of the exercises in the chapter can be done at home in no time at all, and the suggestions can be worked into your lifestyle without major adjustments. Give these guidelines a chance, and you'll notice the difference in how you look and in how you feel.

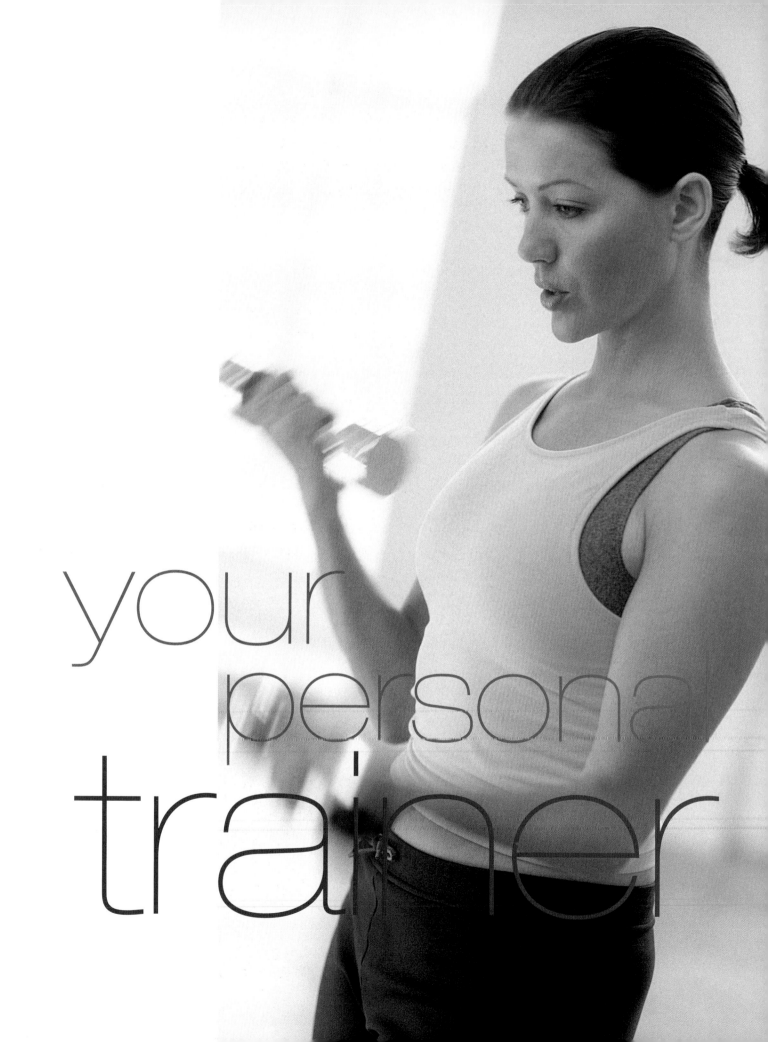

your
personal
trainer

While I've learned a great deal about fitness over the years, I'm not a fitness expert. So to help me put this together, I've turned to someone who is. Greg Durham is a certified personal trainer and has an amazing approach to fitness. He treats each client as an individual and crafts a routine that strengthens body and soul. He's helped me get into shape, and now he's going to help you.

five great reasons to work out

boost your energy. Working out won't sap your strength. You might feel a bit zonked when you start an exercise regimen, but over time you'll feel great and you'll build endurance.

look better in your clothes. Work out for two weeks and your jeans won't be quite as tight and your skirts will become less snug.

fight the blues. If you're prone to depression, you'll find that exercise elevates your mood.

strengthen your bones. Working out with weights helps prevent osteoporosis, a disease in which bones weaken as you get older. Women are especially prone to this disease, but your bones, like your muscles, get stronger when you exercise.

improve your health. I don't know a lot of healthy couch potatoes, do you?

how do you rate?

Answer the following questions.

1. Are you strong?
2. Do you have good endurance?
3. Are you flexible?

If you answered yes to all of them, that's great. You should feel good about yourself and continue to challenge your body and mind with different types of exercise. Or maybe you answered yes to one and no to the others. Maybe you're in pretty sad shape when it comes to all three categories. Don't beat yourself up just yet. We're only getting

En•dor•phins *(n)* The chemicals in your brain that help relieve pain and boost your mood. Exercise is believed to stimulate them.

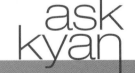

ask kyan

Q. Do I need a personal trainer?

A. A trainer is a real luxury. If you can afford one, that's great. He or she will keep you motivated and devise a routine that's tailored to your needs. If you join a gym, a free training session is usually included. If you already belong but can't afford a trainer, ask the employees for assistance. You also can ask other gym members who look like they're in really good shape. They'll probably be flattered and happy to help.

started. It's good to be honest because you'll understand where you have work to do.

write it down

Go grab a piece of paper and a pen. I want you to make a list of everything you do to stay physically fit. Maybe there are exercises you do that you don't even realize. Do you run up and down stairs 10 times a day? Walk your dog? Chase after your kids? Scribble it all down. If you do nothing, write that down too.

Now I want you to evaluate your list. Are you happy with the amount of exercise that you do? Is there room for improvement? Think back to the physical fitness checklist: strength, endurance, and flexibility. Are you doing enough to achieve all three?

set goals

Now it's time to write down your goals. You don't have to show them to anyone, so make them as personal as you want. Perhaps you're tired all the time and want more energy. Maybe you want to shape up your butt and thighs, look better in a bathing suit, run a marathon, or get into yoga. You can mention any reason under the sun, but it's really important to have some goals in mind because it will help motivate you.

get moving!

If you already have a workout routine, you can jump ahead. This section is for all the workout virgins, couch potatoes, and desk potatoes out there (you know who you are). I bet you have a million excuses—and some of them are probably good ones. I know mine always are! Gyms are expensive, personal trainers are a fortune, the yoga center doesn't offer classes at a convenient hour, your apartment's too small to work out in, there's not enough time in the day, and you're too darn tired. But you know what they say—excuses, excuses.

Don't let excuses rule your life.

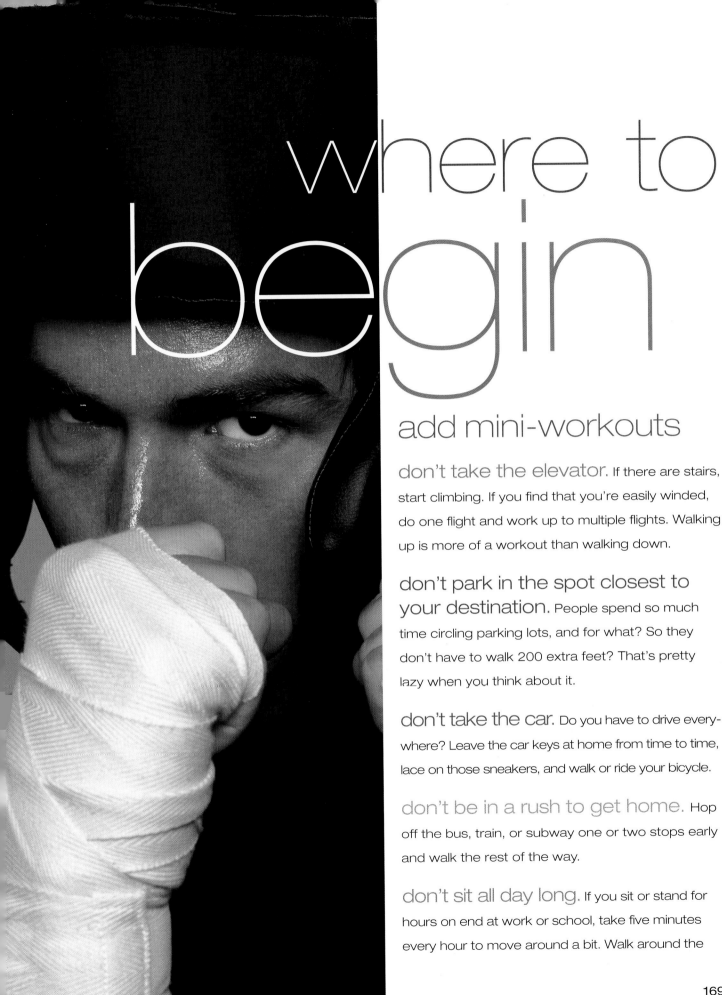

where to begin

add mini-workouts

don't take the elevator. If there are stairs, start climbing. If you find that you're easily winded, do one flight and work up to multiple flights. Walking up is more of a workout than walking down.

don't park in the spot closest to your destination. People spend so much time circling parking lots, and for what? So they don't have to walk 200 extra feet? That's pretty lazy when you think about it.

don't take the car. Do you have to drive everywhere? Leave the car keys at home from time to time, lace on those sneakers, and walk or ride your bicycle.

don't be in a rush to get home. Hop off the bus, train, or subway one or two stops early and walk the rest of the way.

don't sit all day long. If you sit or stand for hours on end at work or school, take five minutes every hour to move around a bit. Walk around the

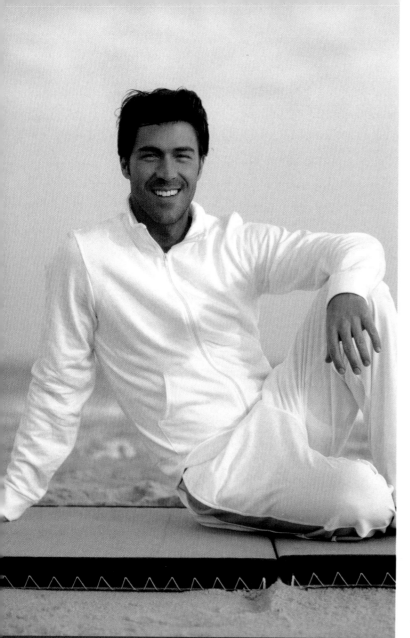

office or the block. Stretch out your arms and your legs. Take long, deep breaths. Rotate your wrists clockwise and counterclockwise, especially if you work on a computer. Roll your shoulders and do light neck rolls, clockwise then counterclockwise. Throughout the day, instead of calling or emailing that colleague down the hall, walk to his or her office.

don't hurt yourself

Whether you're new to working out, or you want to intensify your routine, take it easy. The most common way to injure yourself is by pushing your body too hard in the beginning. You can make your workout more challenging over time, but do it in small increments.

You also want to focus on form. Pay attention to the photos that accompany each exercise in this chapter and go slowly. You never want to rush through a workout. If you feel your form getting sloppy, stop. It's better, for example, to do two push-ups properly than seven mediocre ones. Proper form ensures that the muscles you want to work out are being exercised. Doing an exercise correctly also will help you avoid injury. Learn to differentiate between good pain and bad pain. You should never feel sharp, stabbing pain during a workout. That's a major indicator of a stress or oncoming injury. If you feel pain like this, stop immediately and rest. On the other hand, if your stomach is "burning," for example, during an intense ab session, that's good. It means that your muscles are working hard.

warm up and cool down It's a smart idea to start your workout with five minutes of light walking on a treadmill or some other moderately intense cardio activity. Once your muscles are

what's up, doc?

If you're starting a new fitness regimen, it's a good idea to check in with your doctor and get a clean bill of health. Have your vital statistics taken, including blood pressure, heart rate, weight, and body mass index (we'll talk more about this later in the chapter). In addition to making sure you're in proper working order, you'll have an accurate record of where you are before starting an exercise regimen. This will be helpful to measure against later as your fitness levels improve.

warm, take five minutes for a good overall stretch, focusing on your major muscle groups. Then you can start your official cardio workout or hit the weights.

The best way to cool down is by stretching. Working out, especially with weights, forces muscles to contract, so in order to maintain flexibility and avoid cramping, you should always stretch afterward to help lengthen muscles.

breathing 101

Before you do a single leg lift or jumping jack, let's review how to breathe. I know what you're thinking: "I know how to breathe." But chances are you don't. Breathing properly helps boost your endurance by delivering more oxygen throughout your body, which helps your heart work less and helps your muscles work harder.

Inhale through your nose and feel your abs and chest expand as you fill your lungs with air. Then exhale through your mouth, slowly and steadily. Don't let the air just whoosh out at a high speed. This is what singers, public speakers, and yoga students learn. *You* control your breath, not the other way around. Long, measured inhales and exhales give you energy and allow you to extend your endurance instead of hyperventilating. Being conscious of your breath might seem strange at first, but over time proper breathing will become a habit. If you're one of those people who's huffing and puffing after a few minutes on the treadmill, then this is especially important. A trick to learning breath control is to time yourself. Inhale for a count of 10, then exhale for a count of 10, and incorporate this kind of consciousness in your workout. During exercise, exhale as you're exerting the maximum resistance, which means you should breathe out when you're doing the toughest part of the exercise. Exhale while pushing yourself up when you're doing a push-up or while raising your torso when you're doing a crunch.

tummy tuck

When you work out, you always want to have your stomach sucked in because that helps protect your lower back. Imagine using your abdominal muscles to "pull" your belly button closer to your spine. But don't let this interfere with your breathing.

change it up

When it comes to exercise, a varied approach is best. To get the maximum results for your body and your health, you should establish a routine that includes cardiovascular activities, weight-bearing exercises, and stretching.

kyanism

Get Motivated
Motivation is one of the most important aspects of fitness. Without it, you have no desire to exercise. What I've learned is that motivation will always come and it will always go. There are times when I feel that it's right around the corner . . . but it takes forever to arrive.

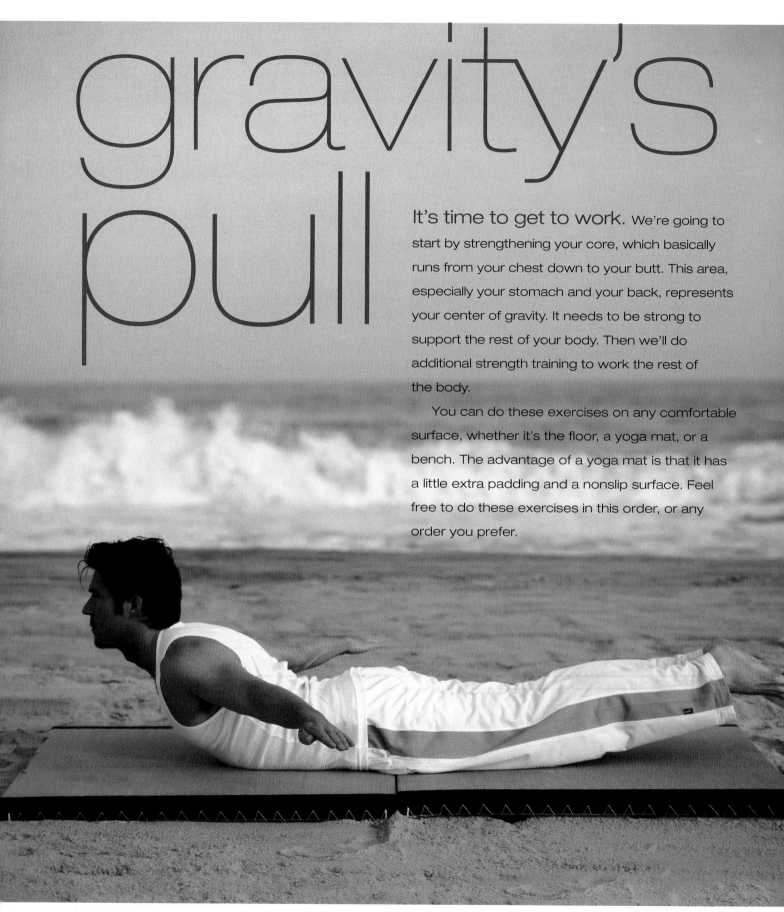

gravity's pull

It's time to get to work. We're going to start by strengthening your core, which basically runs from your chest down to your butt. This area, especially your stomach and your back, represents your center of gravity. It needs to be strong to support the rest of your body. Then we'll do additional strength training to work the rest of the body.

You can do these exercises on any comfortable surface, whether it's the floor, a yoga mat, or a bench. The advantage of a yoga mat is that it has a little extra padding and a nonslip surface. Feel free to do these exercises in this order, or any order you prefer.

the airplane

reps and sets
Every time you do one push-up, one bicep curl, one crunch, or whatever exercise you're performing, that is a rep, which is short for repetition. The number of reps you do before you rest constitutes one set. For the exercises that follow, I suggest you do three sets of each. The number of reps depends on you. Maybe you can do 5, or maybe you can do 12. Don't overexert yourself, but don't wimp out either. Increase the number of reps as you get stronger.

For the resistance exercises with weights, you want to do 3 sets, 8 to 12 reps per set. If you're doing more than 12 reps easily and you want to challenge yourself, it's time for heavier weights. You can adjust the amount of reps and sets depending on your fitness goals and body type.

back strengthening
This is an excellent, all-around back strengthener, especially for the muscles of the lower back. You should feel this from your shoulders all the way down to your butt.

Lie face down on the floor with your legs hip width apart and arms straight out in front of you. Your palms should be facing down.

Lift your chest, arms, and legs as high as you can, without bending your arms or legs, and hold for 10 seconds. As you become stronger, you can increase the time you hold this position—15 seconds, 30 seconds, or 1 minute, up to your degree of comfort. Then lower your arms and legs.

challenge yourself
Once you're comfortable with this exercise, try these variations:

the airplane
Raise your chest, arms, and legs like you did on the previous exercise. Quickly move your arms out to the side like airplane wings, palms to the floor, while keeping your legs on the floor. See if you can raise your chest even higher with your arms in this position. Remember, you hold this pose for as short or as long a period as you're comfortable. As you build your strength and endurance, you'll upgrade your goals.

the bow
This exercise is great for strengthening the lower back, but take it slowly at first if you have lower back problems. Lie face down on the floor. Bend your legs at the knees, grasp your ankles, and pull your feet toward your butt. Raise your feet toward the ceiling and try to lift your thighs off the floor, even just a tiny bit. At the same time, lift your chest. When

kyanism
Fanny Focus So many women concentrate on their butts, stomachs, and thighs and neglect their upper bodies. Don't fall into that trap. Give equal time to your back, arms, and shoulders so that you're fit from head to toe.

you're comfortable in the position, see if you can lift those feet even closer toward the ceiling, using them to further elevate your thighs and chest off the floor. Hold this position for as long as you can.

shoulder bridge This is great for upper thighs, butt, and lower back. You should also feel your abs engaged.

Lie flat on your back with your legs bent, feet on the floor, about a foot from your butt. Let your hands rest on the ground at your sides. Lift your pelvis as high as it will go toward the ceiling. When you're at your max, stop and hold. How long you hold the position is up to you. Start with 10 seconds and gradually build up until you're able to hold it for a few minutes.

crunches Crunches work your entire abdominal complex.

Lie flat on your back, legs bent, with the soles of your feet on the floor about a foot from your butt and your hands behind your head.

Lift your chest toward the ceiling as high off the floor as you can make it. Hold your form and keep your elbows in place.

Lower your back to the floor. Repeat until you max out.

warning! A common mistake is to lift your head and bend your neck toward your chest as you do a crunch. When done correctly, crunches do not require the use of your neck muscles. Keep your neck and shoulders relaxed and don't bend your neck. Use your abdominal muscles to lift your chest.

challenge yourself It's important to do some variations on the basic crunch. Your abdomen consists of many different muscles and the basic crunch only works a few of them.

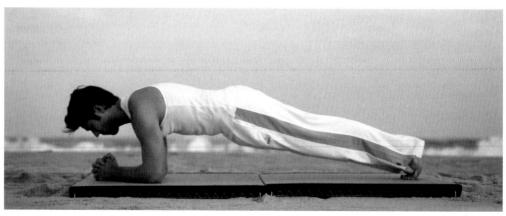

plank

side crunch This is one of the best moves to target your oblique abdominals.

Lie flat on your back, knees bent and pointing toward the ceiling, feet flat on the floor, hands behind your head. Drop your knees to the right. The right knee should be resting on the floor. Your torso will be turned a bit to the side, but both shoulders should be on the floor.

Lift your chest toward the ceiling as high up off the floor as you can make it. Don't turn to the side as you do the crunch. You should move your upper body as though this is a traditional crunch.

Lower your back to the floor. After one set, drop your knees to the left and start over to work the other side.

plank This is one of the best methods of toning your entire core, from the thighs to the torso.

Come into plank position, as though you're ready to do a push-up. Keep your body as straight as a board, from your head to your toes during the entire exercise. Place your forearms flat on the floor and parallel to your body, with your hands in front of you, so that your elbows and forearms are supporting your body. Your elbows, forearms, and toes should be the only parts of your body that are making contact with the floor. Your elbows should be straight below your shoulders and your forearm and biceps should form a 90 degree angle. (Keep your stomach muscles isometrically contracted to protect your back. Never let your stomach sag toward the floor).

Hold for as long as you can without losing your form. Really keep that stomach flexed the entire time.

push-ups This is a great workout for flabby arms.

Come into a push-up position with your hands shoulder-width apart. Visualize yourself as a straight board. Don't let your stomach sink down toward the floor. This is bad form and it puts stress on your lower back. Good form will ensure that your pectoral muscles are doing the work to get you up and down.

Bend your arms and lower yourself to the point where your arms are at a 90-degree angle to the floor. Don't let your elbows splay out too far to the side. If you want to work your triceps more, keep your elbows pinned to your side.

Push yourself back up. Repeat until you max out or until your form starts getting sloppy.

kyanism

I'm Just a Girl How did this guy-girl push-up thing start anyway? Because of it, a lot of girls think they're not strong enough to do a "guy" push-up and don't even try. I want you to try to do at least one guy push-up. Once you've mastered that, try to add another each time you work out. No special treatment, ladies, but if you really can't do one, I'd rather you did "girl" push-ups than none at all.

challenge yourself To really work out those triceps, follow the same directions as above, but move your hands closer together. A super-advanced move is the close-grip push-up, where your hands are side by side.

leg lifts You will feel this in your lower abdominals and hip flexors.

Lie with your back on the floor and arms against your sides, legs straight in front of you or bent at the knee. (If this is too challenging, or bothers your back, place your hands under your butt so they form a little cushion for your bottom.) Remember to pull your belly button toward your spine to protect your lower back. Don't pull with your lower back.

Lift your legs up and down. Keep them straight the entire time and lift until they're at a 90 degree angle to the floor. Do not let your feet touch the ground in between reps. It's important to use controlled motion and a consistent speed during lifts. It should take you the same amount of time to come down that it takes to lift your legs up.

squats This exercise mainly works your thighs and glutes.

Stand with your legs hip width apart, toes facing straight in front of you, and arms at your sides. Suck in your abs.

Lower your butt (pretend you're going to sit in a chair) until your upper thighs are parallel to the floor. At the same time, raise your arms in front of you until they are parallel to the floor. Keep your stomach sucked in and maintain an upright posture. Don't slouch.

Slowly return to the standing position. At the same time, lower your arms to your sides.

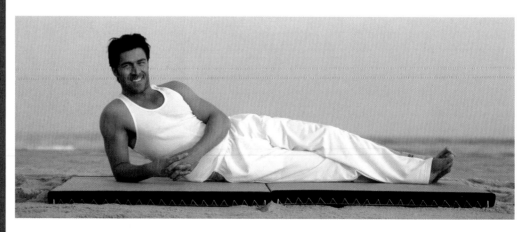

challenge yourself When doing your squats, hold hand weights. This will work your legs, butt, and shoulders at the same time.

the lunge You will feel this burn in your thighs and butt.

Stand with your feet together and toes pointed straight ahead, with your hands on your hips. Take a step backward with the right leg, bending your right knee (but don't let your knee touch the floor).

Your left leg will bend naturally. Lower your body until your left leg bends to about a 90 degree angle with your left thigh parallel to the floor. Slowly return to a standing position, using the strength in your left leg to stand up. Alternate legs.

challenge yourself Hold a weight in each hand while you do the lunges.

heartbeat Let's talk about cardio. You've heard this term before, right? Well, the *cardio*vascular system includes your heart and blood vessels, and cardio refers to any type of exercise that gets your heart revved up—climbing stairs, running, walking, jogging, cleaning your house. By raising your heart rate, you're putting stress on your heart (in a good way) and helping it grow stronger. A stronger heart will pump blood more efficiently.

When you're doing a cardio activity, pick up your pace and see how long you can go until you're out of breath. Each time, increase the intensity some more. When you are starting out, try 10 minutes of walking on a treadmill at a moderate pace and modify as your fitness increases. Depending on your goals (maybe you want to run a marathon?)

you may need to spend more time on cardio. A lot of people think that they need to jump on a treadmill for 45 minutes to get their heart rate up, but they don't. You can do that if you like, but you'll also get your heart rate up from strength training, yoga, or any other strenuous exercise.

take your pulse Exercise is all about raising your heart rate. When you do this for an extended period of time, you're getting fit while building muscle and burning calories and fat. A helpful equation for measuring your heart rate was developed by Dr. Philip Maffetone. Subtract your age from 180. This is your target heart rate during exercise. You want to maintain this, or stay in this range for most of your workout, excluding warm-ups and cool-downs. If you're recovering from an injury or illness, don't be too hard on yourself, though. It's fine to work below this level if you're not feeling your best.

ask kyan

Q. Once I start working out, when will I notice a difference in my body?

A. When I've slacked off and then started exercising again, I've generally noticed a difference after a week. I'm not talking about defined muscles and six-pack abs; rather I start to feel better about myself and have more energy, and I see a slight firming of my muscles. If you're doing a serious workout at least three times a week, you should get the same results. After a few weeks of dedicated exercise, three to five times a week, you should notice that your clothes fit better. If you're working with weights, you might notice a bit of definition after a month.

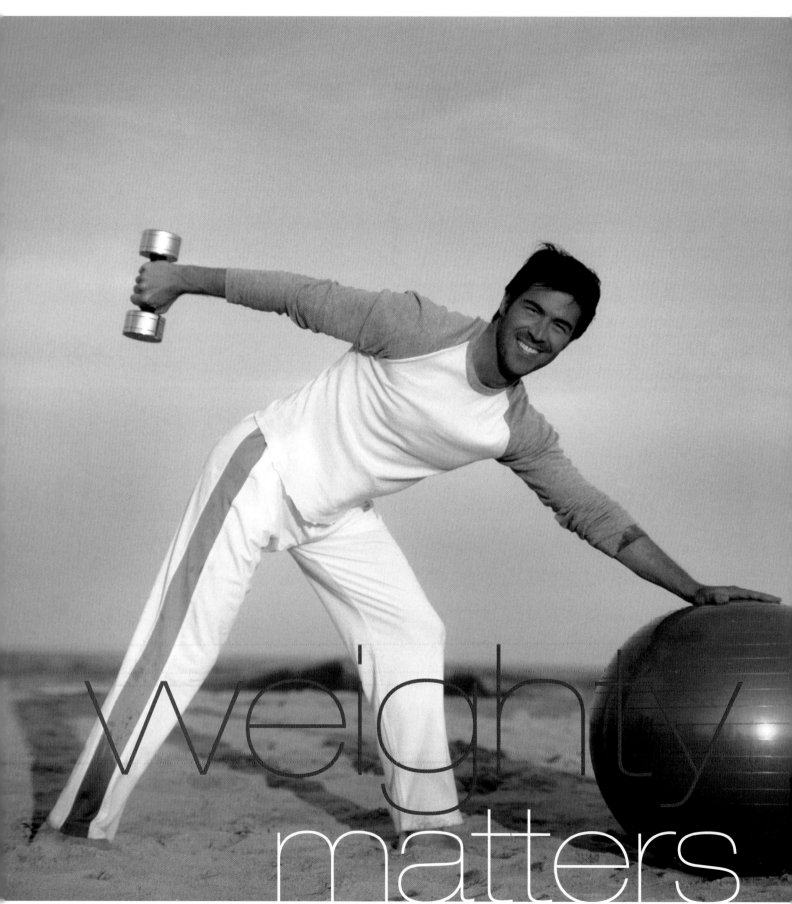

Weighty
matters

tricep pushback

You should have a few sets of hand weights for the exercises in this section. A set you can lift 8 to 10 times is ideal, plus another set that's a few pounds heavier. When you're at the store, do a bicep curl and test the weight before you buy. Upgrade to the heavier weights when the lighter ones no longer present a challenge.

bicep curl This is a great overall strengthener for your biceps.

Stand up straight, arms at your sides, and hold the weights with your palms facing forward. With your elbows pinned to your sides, bend your arm and pull the weight toward your shoulder. The only things you should be moving are your forearms.

tricep pushback If weak triceps are an issue, focus on this workout. Get a hard chair, like a wood or metal one you'd find at a kitchen table. (You can also use a Swiss ball.) Put your left knee on the seat of the chair, and your left hand on the back of the chair. Lean your upper body toward the chair so that your body is at a 45 degree angle to the floor. The chair should stay on the floor at all times. This is the starting position.

Hold a weight in your right hand and bend your arm back, so that your upper arm (triceps) is parallel to the floor, and your forearm is perpendicular to the floor. Think of your upper arm as an unmoving part of a machine with the elbow as its axis. This part of your arm should never move during the exercise. Keeping your elbow close to your side, push your forearm back and up until your arm is straight. Lower your forearm to the starting position and then continue for as many reps as possible.

Alternate sides for a second set.

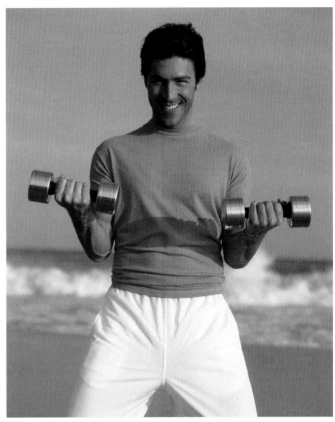

bicep curl

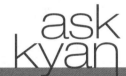

Q. A lot of people at my gym talk about their body-fat percentage. What are they referring to?

A. Your body-fat percentage is literally how much fat your body holds. There are different ways to gauge it. Your doctor can do a skin-fold measurement (or pinch test) with calipers, or it can also be gauged with bioelectric impedance analysis (BIA), where a painless electric current is sent through the body. Neither test is 100 percent accurate. You might also hear people talk about body mass index, or BMI. This is an estimation of your total body fat based on your height to weight ratio. If your body fat percentage is too high, it can mean that you're obese, which puts you at risk for cancer, high blood pressure, and heart disease. It's in your best interest to start eating right and working out to get those numbers down.

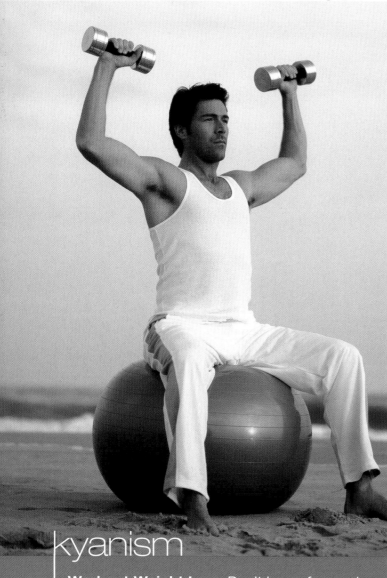

kyanism

Workout Weight Loss Don't be so focused on weight loss. Even if you've been working out steadily for a month, because muscle weighs more than fat, you won't notice a drastic change when you step on the scale. In fact, throw away your scale. A better way to measure your progress is with a fabric tape measure. Record the circumference of your arms, waist, hips, and thighs, then check your progress every few weeks. In any case, don't become obsessed with your weight or measurements. It's easy to become a slave to numbers.

military press You'll really feel your shoulder muscles working here.

Sit in a chair with your knees bent at a 90 degree angle and your feet flat on the floor. Hold your weights in each hand and, bending at your elbows, lift your arms out to your sides until your triceps are parallel to the floor and your forearms are perpendicular to the ceiling, with your weights pointed toward the ceiling. This is the starting position.

Lift your arms toward the ceiling in a controlled motion, touching the weights together above your head. Don't attempt to straighten completely (your elbows should never lock during this exercise). Slowly bring the weights back down to the starting position. Do as many reps as possible.

bench press

This push-up in reverse really works your pectorals and your triceps.

Lie on your back, legs flat or bent, weights in each hand, elbows against your sides, and forearms at a 90 degree angle with the floor. This is the starting position.

Push the weights toward the ceiling. You also can touch the weights together and hold for a second. Don't lock your elbows. Your arms should be almost straightened, but not quite.

Lower your arms back down to the starting position. Do as many reps as possible.

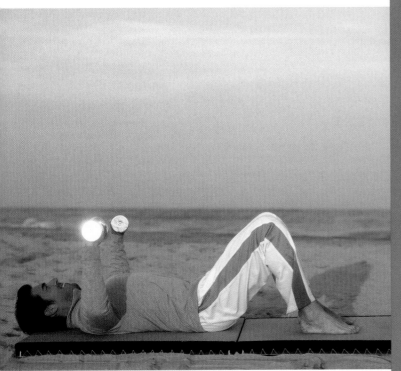

bench press

super set

Let's say you're working with a 10-pound set of dumbbells and you're exhausted after seven reps. Pick up whatever lighter dumbbell you have around and do two or three more reps with that. You'll increase your strength by challenging your muscles this way.

change will do you good
Don't get bored by your routine. Change it up from time to time. If you don't vary your routine, you'll find that you're less interested and less challenged. Your muscles are smarter than you think! They'll find ways to adapt to the same workout.

fitness fashion

Are you worried that you don't have the right sneakers or the little velour sweatsuit that everybody else does? You shouldn't think about your workout as a fashion show, but who am I kidding? The gym, yoga class, or local jogging path is a great place to meet people, so there's nothing wrong with wanting to look your best. Personally, I dress for comfort, but for some people, buying cool workout clothes (your "gym drag," as I like to call it) and wearing them is a real motivator. That said, don't get overly focused on what's cute.

You want to wear clothes that are functional, comfortable, and breathable. You don't want anything too baggy when you're doing strength training or yoga, or it will get in the way. If you're self-conscious, dress in a way that's going to make you feel better if that's what it takes to get you to the gym. Wear a loose T-shirt and cargo pants. Who cares?

Your shoes are the most important aspect of your workout wardrobe. If your feet hurt, it's hard to get motivated. Make sure your sneakers fit well and provide arch support.

kyanism

Muscle Myths I know you want to look toned, not muscled. There's no way you're going to look like a professional wrestler following the exercises in this book. For that, you'll need an intense weight-training program.

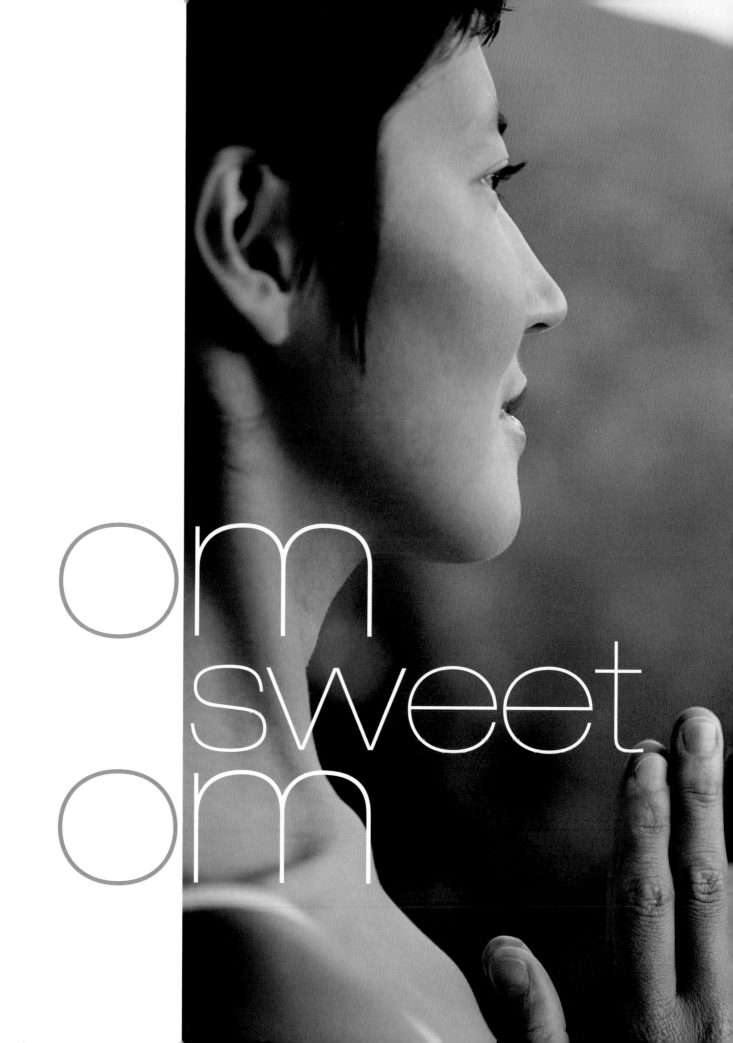

om
sweet
om

If you haven't been turned on to yoga yet, it's time. You don't know what you're missing. Not only is it a great way to increase your flexibility, it also strengthens your body, raises your heart rate, calms your mind, and gets you in touch with your spirit—all at once. I can't think of another exercise that makes the mind-body-spirit connection so powerfully.

The actual practice of yoga involves moving your body through a series of poses, meditative breathing, and chanting. There are dozens of types of yoga practiced today; some are steeped in tradition alone, no frills; some are rather trendy. The main differences generally have to do with the sequence in which the poses are done and at what pace and intensity. But they're all centered around a common philosophy of learning how to breathe so that it relaxes your body and mind. The more relaxed you are, the more flexible you can become.

Don't view yoga as a competition. You should feel comfortable going at your own pace and pushing yourself as much or as little as you want. Just because someone else in the class seems more advanced, don't feel the need to keep up with him or her.

Your instructor probably will ask if there are any beginners in the room. If it's your first class, don't be embarrassed to raise your hand. This way, the instructor will pay more attention to you and check on your form from time to time. (If you're new to yoga, be aware that no one wears shoes or socks during the class. Take care of those dirty soles and grungy toes before leaving the house!)

Yoga gives you an opportunity to recognize the negative patterns in your life. If you tend to blame others, you'll probably want to blame your instructor for not explaining things correctly or holding poses for too long. If you tend to beat yourself up, you'll get critical when you can't do certain poses. Be open enough and patient enough to realize what you're doing and work through it.

yoga 101

Here are the most common types of yoga practiced today:

hatha (pronounced hah-thuh) A beginner's Hatha class is a great place to start if you're new to yoga. You'll learn the basic postures and breathing techniques that form the basis of all other forms of yoga.

ashtanga (pronounced ahsh-ton-ga) Also known as power yoga, this is great if you're already familiar with the basic yoga postures and you're looking for a more intense workout.

kyanism

Yucky Yoga Mats If you commit to yoga, it's a good idea to buy your own mat. Otherwise, you might have to rent one every time you take a class. But don't ruin your karma with a dirty yoga mat. Keep yours clean by sticking it in the tub and washing with some soap or mild detergent after class. Throw it over the shower rod to dry.

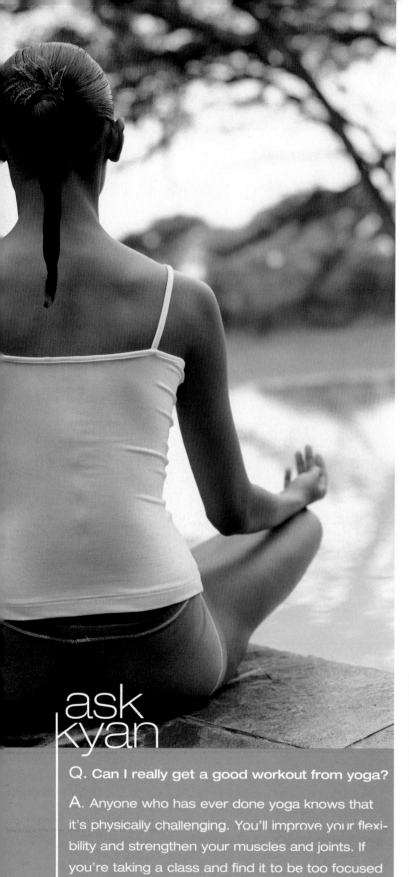

iyengar (pronounced eye-en-gar)

This is more meditative than Ashtanga. The precision of the poses is a big focus of Iyengar.

bikram (pronounced bick-rahm) This

is performed in a room that's heated to 104°F. The belief is that the warmer your body is, the deeper you can go into the poses. Muscles love heat, and the warmer they are, the more relaxed they are.

pilates

This type of exercise, or "method," as it's called, was developed decades ago by a man named Joseph Pilates. It revolves around a series of exercises you do on the floor (often referred to as mat work) or on machines (which have names like the Reformer and Cadillac). It's a great workout because it combines strength training, raising your heart rate, and improving your flexibility.

Unlike yoga, Pilates is strictly geared toward working those core muscles that will give you a strong body. Like yoga, you're focused on your breathing during Pilates, so you get into that Zen frame of mind. It's very meditative because your mind clears as you focus solely on the exercise at hand.

ask kyan

Q. Can I really get a good workout from yoga?

A. Anyone who has ever done yoga knows that it's physically challenging. You'll improve your flexibility and strengthen your muscles and joints. If you're taking a class and find it to be too focused on the meditative side of things, consider more athletic forms, such as Bikram or Ashtanga. If you're skeptical about the athleticism involved in yoga, you'll get your butt kicked in these classes.

budget workout

If money's tight, don't worry. You don't need a gym membership, a personal trainer, fancy clothes, or equipment to get in shape. It doesn't cost a thing to go for a walk, climb up and down a few flights of stairs, or do a series of crunches and push-ups. In fact, none of the core exercises we discussed earlier requires anything except sneakers. If you're curious about yoga or Pilates, borrow some books or tapes from the library and teach yourself the basics.

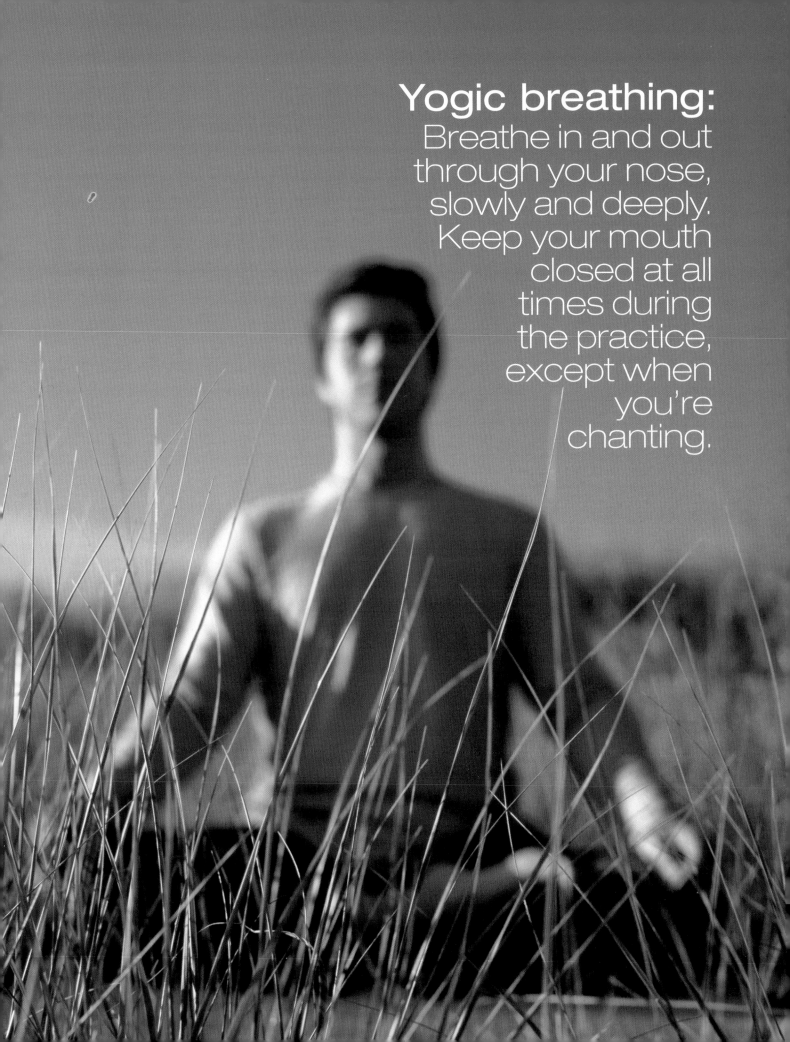

Yogic breathing:
Breathe in and out through your nose, slowly and deeply. Keep your mouth closed at all times during the practice, except when you're chanting.

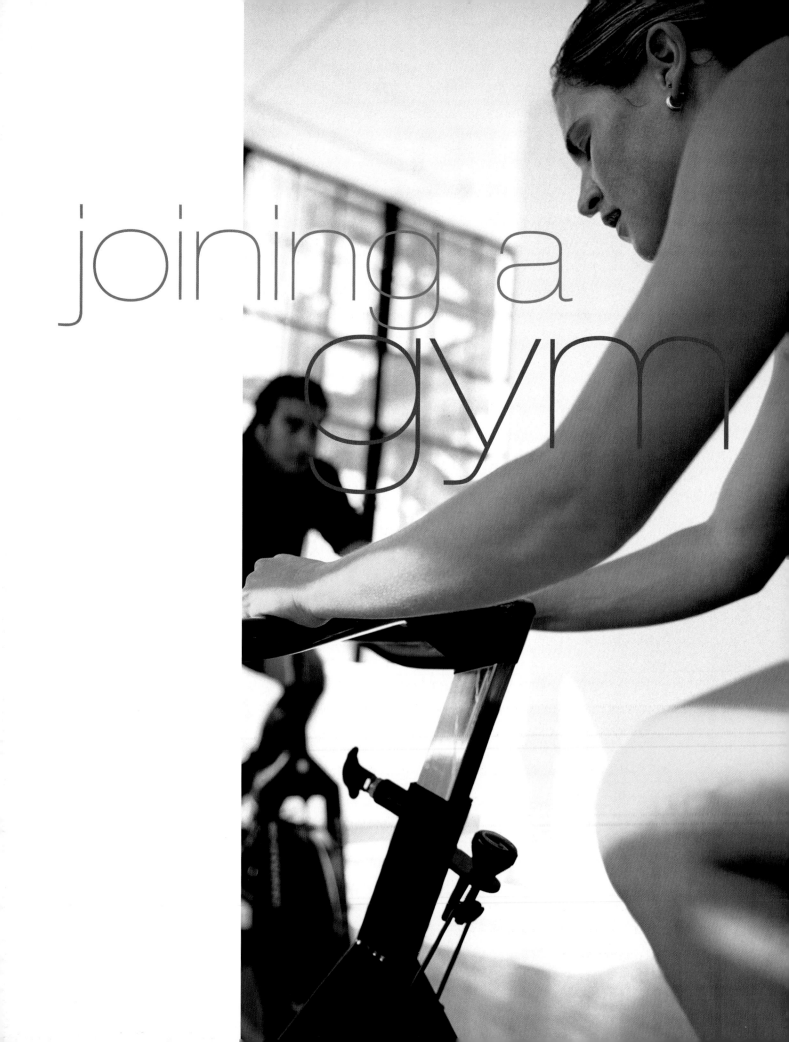

joining a
gym

Nothing beats a gym. There are great classes and terrific equipment; cute, buff members to keep you motivated; nice showers and maybe a steam room and sauna. The key to getting the most from your membership? Taking advantage of what your gym has to offer. Don't know how to use a certain piece of equipment? Find an employee or another member and ask for a demonstration. Don't be shy. The same goes for classes. Try a few until you find one that you like. Ask the instructor for help or pointers before, during, or after the class. If a free training session is included in your membership, use it. If not, ask if the club will throw one in.

Here are a few of the classes your gym might offer.

body sculpting Tighten, tone, and condition using different pieces of equipment, like weights, bands, and bars.

kickboxing Different drills and fundamentals of the sport are taught. You'll get a good cardio workout while improving your agility and quickness.

gyrotonics You work your spine, muscles, and joints on a special piece of equipment consisting of weights, pulleys, and wheels. Great for flexibility and toning.

core fusion (or core conditioning) Strengthen and define your abdominals and other core muscles through a variety of floor exercises.

spinning This is a cardio workout done on a stationary bicycle. Since you're in control of the bike's resistance, you can make the workout as challenging as you want. Great for beginners and nonbeginners alike.

step aerobics This features choreographed exercises using a "step," which is essentially a sturdy box that you step on or over during the exercises.

Of course, once you join a gym, you have to actually show up. You'd be amazed how many people pay each month to keep their membership active and never go. They think they're one step closer to being fit by virtue of that membership. If that's you, cancel your membership right now! It's just another thing to feel guilty about. Work out at home and join again when you're ready to make a real commitment.

kyanism

Social Shape-up
Try incorporating fitness into your social life. Don't rely on your friends to get your workout in gear, but suggest going for a walk instead of getting a drink, or take a yoga class together and then get a healthy lunch afterward. Realize that incorporating fitness and time with your friends is fun and healthy. It's a great way to connect with others and take care of yourself simultaneously.

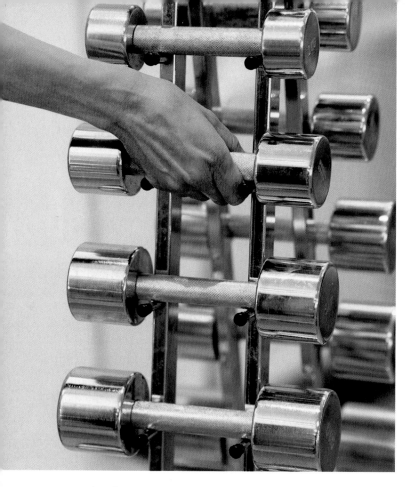

at-home gym

No time to work out? Too beat to get to the gym? Bring the gym to you. You don't need to spend a lot of money to outfit your house or apartment, unless you're really into working out and you want to invest in some machines.

Here are some basics to have:

handweights
Buy a few sets if you can afford it. Start with something you can lift 8 to 12 times without getting exhausted.

exercise bands
These are giant rubberbands that let you do a range of resistance exercises. The elasticity is great for people with joint issues.

jump rope
Everybody knows how to use a jump rope. You'll really get your heart pumping and burn a lot of calories if you do a cardio workout with this.

stability ball
Also know as a Swiss ball, this is great for strengthening your core muscles and improving your posture. You can sit on it while you watch TV or work on your computer, or incorporate it into certain workouts.

floor mat
Any kind of mat, like a yoga mat, will do. You want something that won't slide around and that will cushion your back.

fuel for your body

Don't exercise on an empty stomach.
Your body is very clever. It's going to use the protein in your muscles as fuel if there's nothing else available. I'm not saying you should sit down to a full meal before a workout, but have a piece of fruit or a bowl of cereal first. Bananas are great because they're easily digestible. I'm not a big fan of protein or carb bars, unless you don't have access to anything else.

Always make sure you have enough water and drink it throughout your workout. Sports drinks are fine, but they're no replacement for water.

SUPER BERRY SMOOTHIE

Here's a recipe for one of my favorite pre-workout mini-meals.

  1 chopped frozen banana
  1 cup frozen mixed berries
    Enough soy or rice milk (or low-fat or skim milk) to properly blend
  1 serving scoop soy protein powder

Put all the ingredients in a blender and mix at high speed. Pour into a glass and enjoy.

keep motivated

To get my motivation moving, I try to find people who inspire me because they're in such good shape. Pick somebody who's a little older than you. It's always sobering when you see somebody 20 years older who could kick your butt.

Another great motivator is music. Let's face it, working out can be boring sometimes. Your favorite tunes will get you into the groove.

Lastly, don't let negative self-talk bring you down. Thinking that I can't do something or reinforcing a negative feeling about a certain body part makes me feel bad about myself. I don't want to do anything except pull the covers over my head and hide. Rather than emphasize what's wrong, I try to focus on what I like about my body and accept those parts of me that aren't perfect. You might not be as thin or as toned as you like, but your body still does some amazing things. If you can change your mind-set just a bit in this direction, it might be a lot easier to summon that motivation.

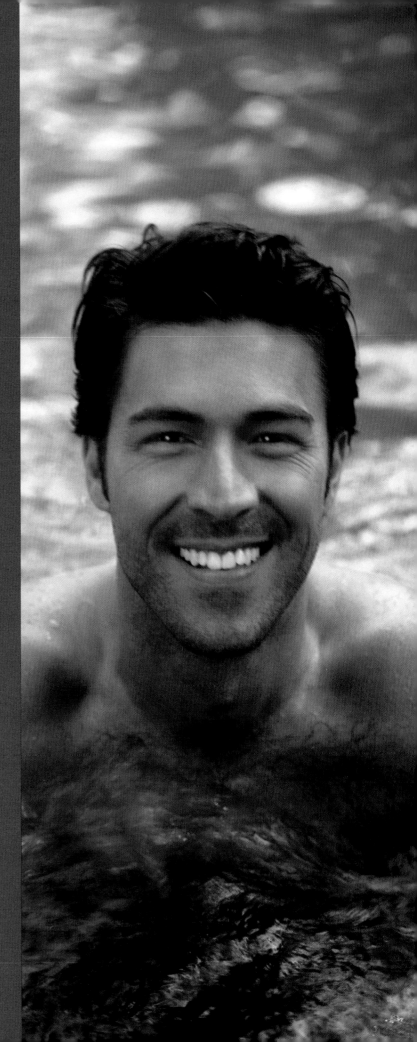

your
spirit
workout

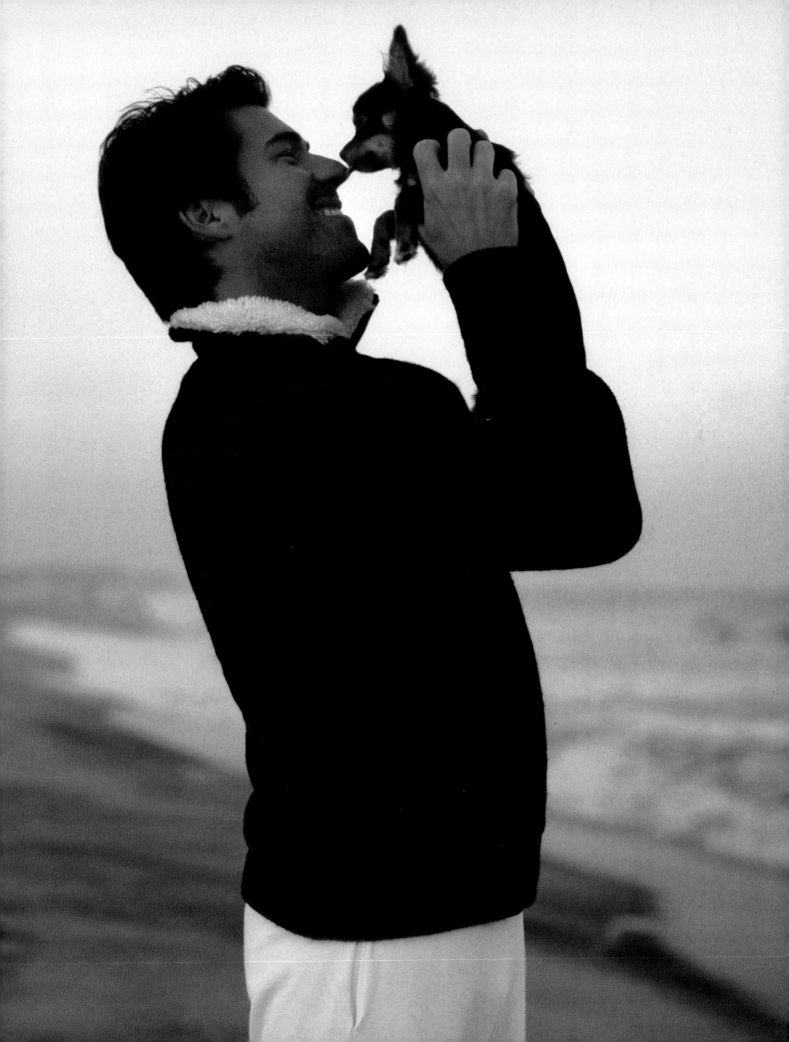

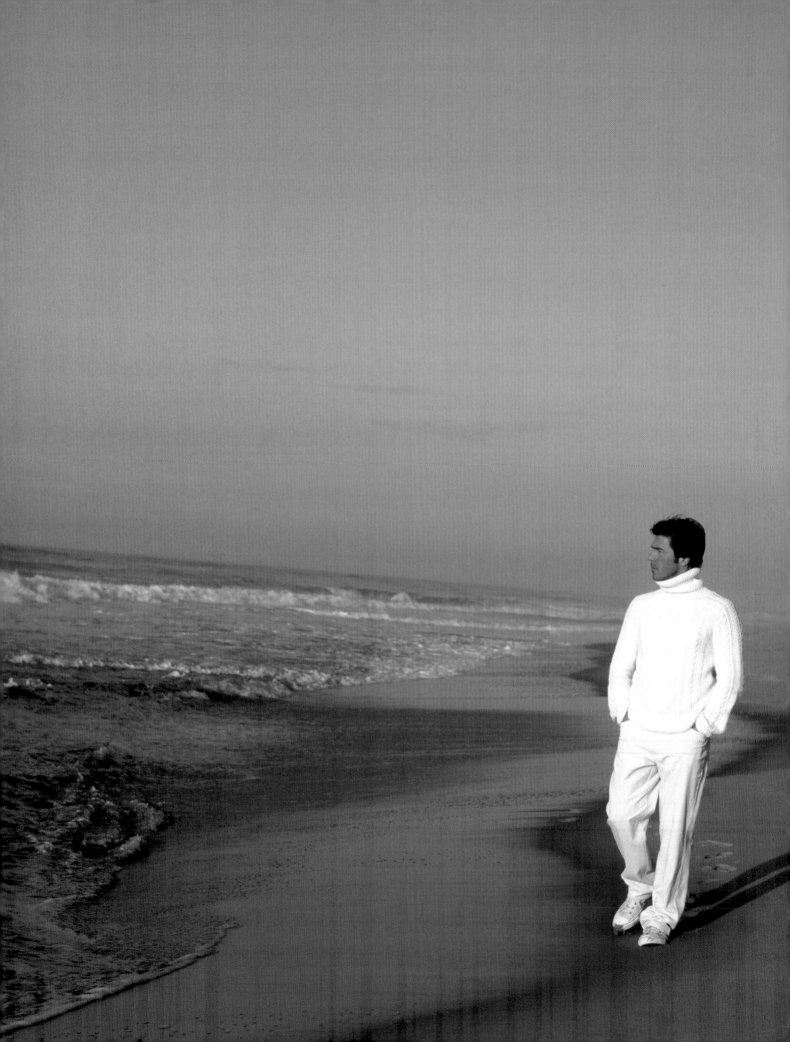

You might think this sounds crazy, but in many ways, your spirit is no different than your abs or your hair or your skin. You need to get it into shape and maintain it. We're talking pretty on the inside. This doesn't just happen, people. It's something you need to consciously work on. Remember, that's what beautified is all about: looking your best, head to toe, inside and out, because you made it happen. You put the effort into it and got results.

Let's talk about the word *spirit* for a second. For a lot of people this is a heavy word with religious connotations, not to be discussed outside of a church, synagogue, mosque, or other place of worship. But for me, your spirit is the sum total of who you are. It's everything we've discussed so far, and then some. It's your life and your surroundings, your friends and your family; it's your religion if you have one; it's your outlook, your attitude, your values, you name it. Being spiritual means taking the time to reflect on who you are and striving to make the world around you a better place.

Even if you're eating well, working out, and following the beauty regimens and guidelines in this book, you still need to devote time to your spirit. Because spiritual development is a very personal experience, it's tough to quantify and can be very challenging. Know that you'll need to create your own path for your spiritual development. Cultivating your spirit is integral to the process to being beautified, and it's well worth it. Developing your spirituality is a perpetual work in process, and if you accept that from the start, you'll be able to work on it without feeling any pressure or sense of urgency. Your spirituality is one of those components that makes you *you*, and this aspect of becoming beautified really is a special and unique process for every person.

I don't know if I've answered what spirit is. I don't know if anyone can define it. But the mystery is part of the whole spiritual development exercise. What you consider spirituality is a very personal thing and by having that conversation with yourself, you might find some answers.

What I do know is that most people neglect their spirit. It's like a muscle you never exercise because you didn't know that you could. Here are some spirited ways to do it.

kyanism

What Surrounds You

One way to work on the inside is to focus on the outside. I'm not talking about your face, body, or hair, but the external world, the physical environment around you. Anything you can do to create a nurturing, positive space for yourself is a terrific tool.

cut the clutter

Nothing gets in your way spiritually and physically like clutter. There's an ancient Chinese practice called feng shui (pronounced fung schway) that is designed to enable you to live in harmony with your surroundings. One of the first rules is to get rid of clutter because it represents trapped energy. I try to keep all my stuff to a minimum, but it's hard. (You'd die if you saw all the beauty products in my apartment.) Still, I have a few tips for triumphing over your pack-rat tendencies.

stop making piles.

Bills, magazines, laundry, dirty dishes. Are you surrounded? For some people, making piles is an instinctive response or an addiction. Once you realize this, you can catch yourself in the act and modify your behavior—take action on those items, instead of letting them pike up (literally) for later.

ransack your closet.

If your clothes are schmushed (I know that's not a word, but you know what I mean), you need to get rid of some stuff. It's always painful to part with clothes and shoes and accessories, but you're not doing yourself or your wardrobe any favors if everything is crushed and wrinkled and impossible to reach.

donate, donate, donate.

Go through your closets, drawers, bookcases, basement, attic, whatever, and donate at least 20 items to a local charity. Not only have you done a good thing for yourself and someone else, you might be able to deduct the value of the goods from your taxes.

a rich life

While we're on this subject, I hope you realize that leading a full life has nothing to do with money. Sure, it would be nice to be rich, but it's not the be all and end all. Believe me, it sounds like a cliché, but there are lots of miserable millionaires out there who have learned that money does not equal happiness.

Remember this—at the end of the day, there will always be someone richer than you and poorer than you. Learn to live within your means and learn how to save. I saw a sign at a bank once that read, "It's not what you make; it's what you save." Wise words, no?

your home is your palace

Not feeling like a king or queen lately? Let's go back to the subject of your surroundings. If you're not comfortable in your home or at your office, you're missing a real opportunity. These places say so much about you. My grandmother certainly knew that. My mother knew that. They kept their houses immaculate because they knew their homes were a reflection of them.

I know you're trying to deal with the clutter. That's a great first step. Now let's talk about other things you can do to make your surroundings truly special.

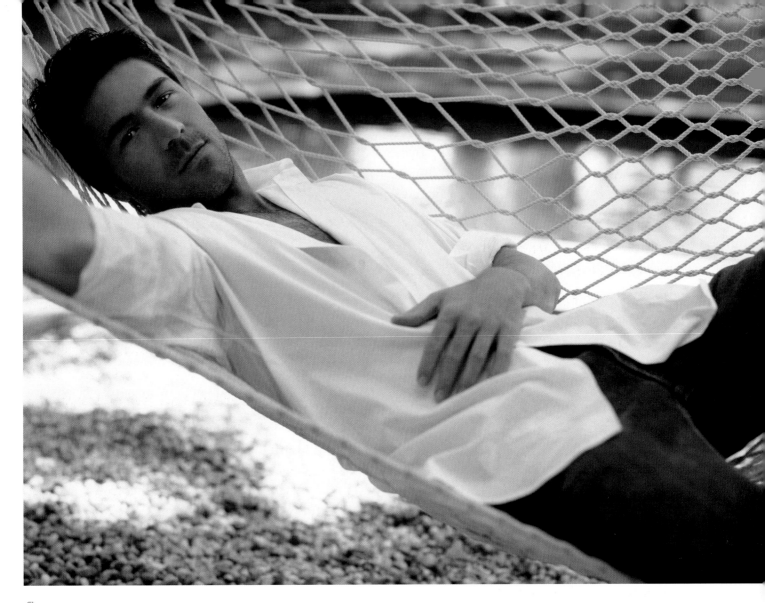

flowers There's a flower market right across the street from my apartment, and I've gotten into the habit of picking out flowers on a regular basis. I tell my boyfriend they're for him, but they're for me, too. You don't need to put them in something fancy. A simple inexpensive vase or wine carafe will do just fine.

lighting This is one of the most important things you can address to alter your space. Do you have lots of stark overhead lighting? That's useful for when you want to vacuum, but that's about it. I much prefer floor lamps, table lamps, sconces, and natural light. They add dimension and depth.

feng shui Maybe you've tried all the things listed here and your home still doesn't feel quite right. This would be a great time for you to investigate feng shui as a framework for remaking your space. There are lots of books and websites on the subject, so you can learn more about the practice. It's okay if you're not very creative when it comes to arranging your furniture. Feng shui offers specific guidelines for designing a room.

kyanism

Make a Living Don't be afraid to try these suggestions at work. You probably spend as many waking hours at the office as you do at home, so make the most of it.

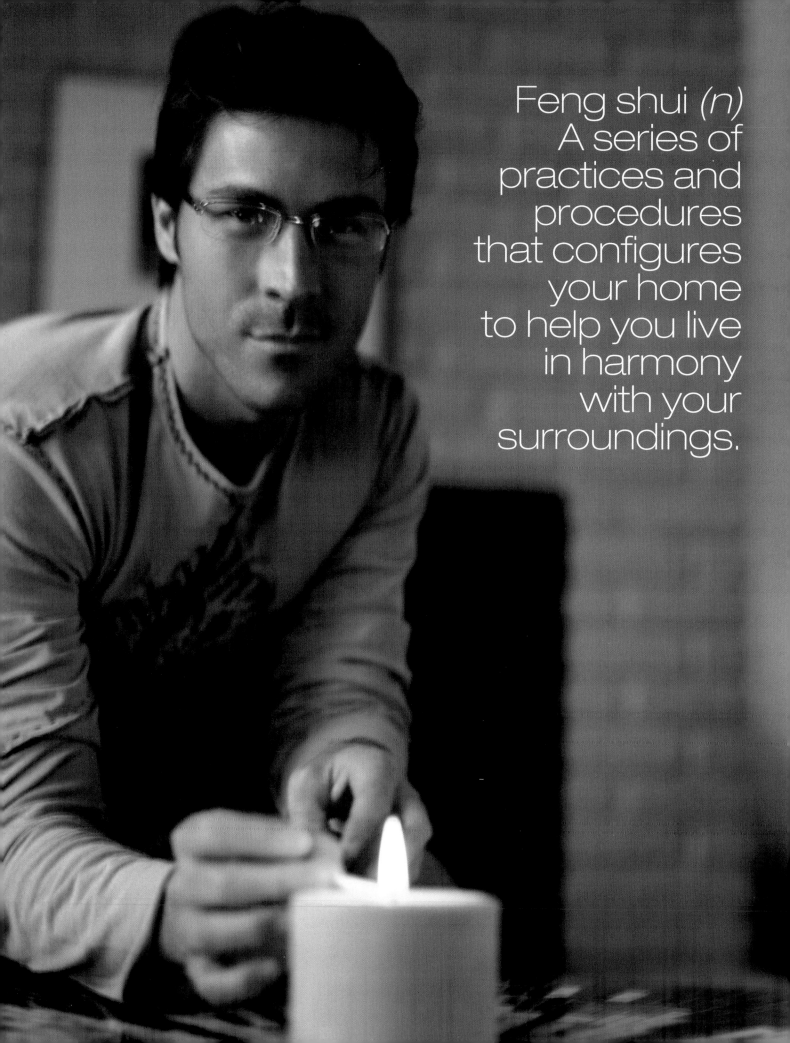

Feng shui (n)
A series of
practices and
procedures
that configures
your home
to help you live
in harmony
with your
surroundings.

candles This is Part B of the lighting lesson. Candles make a room feel sexy and special because they create an instant intimacy and bring an immediate warmth to any space. I like to light several unscented candles and just one scented candle. Too many scented candles will compete with one another and overwhelm your nose. Small votive candles are great and look best in bunches. Buy a dozen and put them in a row, or cluster them in a few different areas.

Trim the wick before you light your candle. It doesn't need to be any longer than a quarter-inch. This way, it will burn evenly, the flame will remain at the proper height, and the room won't get smoky.

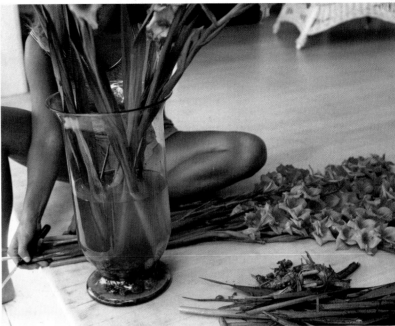

incense If candles aren't your thing, incense is a great way to scent and purify your surroundings. Plus, aroma is really underappreciated as a tool for evoking a mood. Avoid incense that smells like fake kiwi or strawberry or some other fruit. Rather, look for incense made from natural essences.

plants Bringing the outdoors inside adds depth, intensity, and warmth to a room. The color of plants is soothing to the eye, and the presence of another living thing adds a level of comfort. If you have a black thumb rather than a green thumb, don't worry. Go to a store where plants are sold and ask for the sturdiest specimen. Find out what kind of light it requires and how much watering. Focus on your ficus or your fern and notice how good it feels to take care of something else.

arts and crafts Is there any art in your home? I always find it really sad when I go to someone's place and they don't have a single painting, poster, or photo anywhere. Art is so inspiring and thought-provoking, it should be a part of everyone's life. People often make the mistake of thinking that they can't afford art. Of course, 99.9 percent of us can't buy a real Picasso or Monet, but we can certainly buy a reproduction of their work. Better yet . . .

. . . Pick up a cool poster at a museum.

. . . Go to an art fair and buy something inexpensive from a local artist.

. . . Enlarge and frame a photo that you or a friend has taken.

. . . Frame a drawing by a young child. There's something so genuine about a simple crayon drawing or fingerpainting.

kyanism

It's Just Stuff You'll feel so much lighter in every way if you get rid of a few things. We live in a very acquisitive world where too often people are measured by their possessions. We're obsessed with stuff. Measure yourself by who you are, not by what you have.

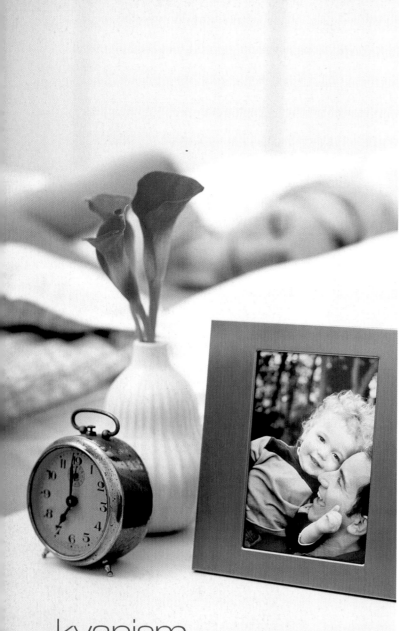

kyanism

Watt Did You Say? Do you really need a high-wattage bulb in every light fixture? Don't trade up. Trade down. It's a good idea to have bright light in your kitchen and any light you use to read or apply makeup by, but try a softer wattage in your other light fixtures. Another thing you can try is one of those pastel light-bulbs. Depending on the color you buy, it will cast a soft, radiant glow over everybody and everything. Also, dimmers can be added to existing lighting fixtures to give you options in creating atmosphere. Think flattering, not floodlight.

photos Don't hide your favorite pictures in scrapbooks. Display them! Pictures of the people, places, even pets that we love are powerful reminders of what matters in life. It's great to be surrounded by the ones we care about, even if they're present in spirit only. Old family photos are great, too. They're a way to honor those who came before us.

hobbies Don't hide your interests in the closet. Find clever ways to incorporate your hobbies into your décor. Your space needs to be reflective of who you are.

color therapy

I have a few questions for you.

- What color are the walls in your bedroom and why?
- What colors are you wearing right now?
- What colors depress you?
- What colors instantly cheer you up?
- Do you have a favorite color?
- What's your favorite lipstick color?

Chances are, you've never given serious thought to these questions. Color is a powerful force, yet we rarely consider its impact on our psyche.

I practice a certain type of color therapy in my apartment. I want my space to provide a sense of comfort and privacy, and I want it to feel like a reward to come home after a long day of work, so I chose luxurious colors for the paint on the walls. Some are a deep, deep chocolate brown, others are light brown, and there's a red-orange shade on my bedroom wall.

Are your walls white or beige? There's nothing wrong with that, provided there are other accents of color throughout your living space. If you want to add some life and vibrancy, consider painting with special colors. Go to the paint store and look at all the color cards. Take some home and see which shades resonate with you. If you fall in love with a color but painting is too much of a hassle, incorporate the color in other ways. Buy some pillows, or a blanket you can throw over a chair, or a small area rug in your favorite shade.

chakras

It makes perfect sense to me that our bodies have concentrations of energy (chakras) and there are ways of channeling or summoning that energy. If you feel that any of your chakras needs fine-tuning, meditate on the corresponding color or bring that color into your life.

- Crown (white): Light and spirituality
- Third Eye (purple): Intuition
- Throat (blue): Communication
- Heart (green): Giving and receiving love
- Solar Plexus (yellow): Relationships and trust
- Spleen (orange): Emotion (sometimes this is referred to as the second chakra)
- Root (red): Strength and passion

Let's say you're having problems communicating. That would mean your throat chakra is blocked. Try focusing on the color blue. Stare at the sky, imagine that color in your head, or wear an article of blue clothing.

This might sound too simplistic to make a difference, but I don't think it is. It's practical and powerful. Do you ever wonder why you choose to wear certain colors each day? Why did you wear white today? Or why did you reach for that red shirt that makes you feel smart or sexy? It's rarely a conscious decision. It's your spirit craving those colors.

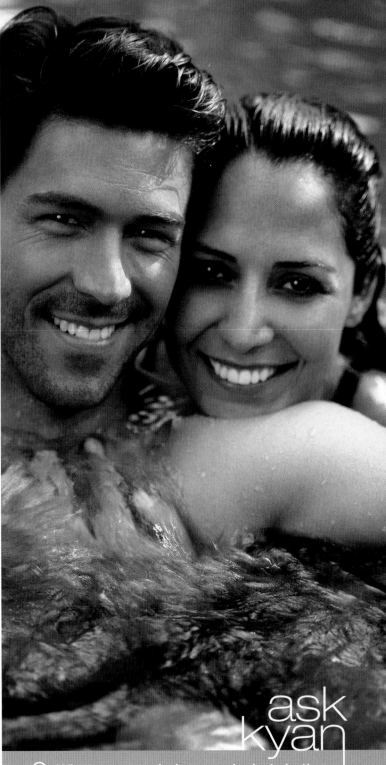

ask kyan

Q. What are my chakras and what do they have to do with color?

A. Inspired by yoga philosophy and pronounced shock-ruhs, chakras are energy centers in our body that have different vibrational frequencies. The vibrations correspond to specific colors, feelings, and emotions. When your chakras are in balance, so is your spirit. By focusing on a certain chakra color, you can affect that energy center.

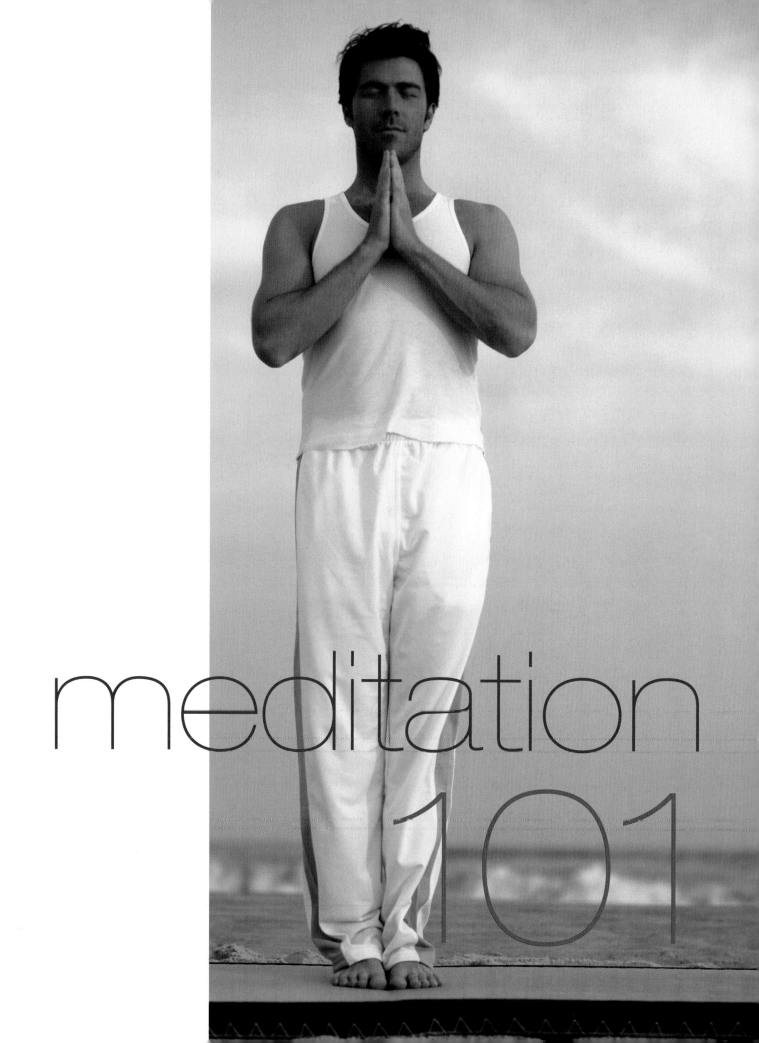

meditation

101

Meditation is awesome. If you've never tried it, you'll love the focus and the clarity it brings to your mind. I'm going to share with you the different kinds of meditation that I practice. First, there's formal, seated meditation where I get into a certain posture (usually the lotus position from yoga, where I'm seated on the floor with my knees touching the ground and my ankles crossed) and consciously focus on my breath for half an hour with the intention of clearing my mind and being completely centered in the moment. You want to suspend thought and just "be." The room is silent except for the sound of my breathing and my eyes are closed. (It might help if you dim the lights, but don't fall asleep!)

The first time you try this, you'll find that your mind doesn't like to be cleared. Your head will be filled with all sorts of random thoughts and visuals, but just focus and breathe. A good way to get rid of all the mental junk is with a mantra. Say it out loud, or you can say it in your head. There's a great Buddhist teacher who suggests a very simple mantra: Say "I know that I am breathing in" as you breath in, and "I know that I am breathing out" as you breath out. See if this works for you.

Another kind of meditation is living in the moment, where you meditate on what you're doing that very second. Whether I'm washing my dishes or brushing my teeth, I focus on bringing awareness to the task at hand. How many times do you mindlessly engage in activities while multitasking or thinking of a million different things at once? I bet this happens all the time. Let's say you're walking in a park. How do your shoes feel on the sidewalk or on the grass? Do you feel the wind in your hair or the sun on the back of your neck? Do you hear birds chirping, cars passing, or kids playing? Think of yourself as being open to everything and sensitive to your surroundings.

breathing basics In the
fitness chapter, we talked about the importance of breathing properly during workouts. Same holds true for meditation. Control of your breath is key. Each time you inhale and exhale, it should be a long, measured, precise action.

ask kyan

Q. I'm so busy I can't find the time to meditate. Does it really make a difference?

A. For me it does. Believe me, I know how hectic the day-to-day can be. But I've found that meditating even for just a little while every day helps me concentrate and focus on my work and responsibilities, and it helps me to stay centered and see things in perspective. It's worth the time because it makes the rest of the day so much better.

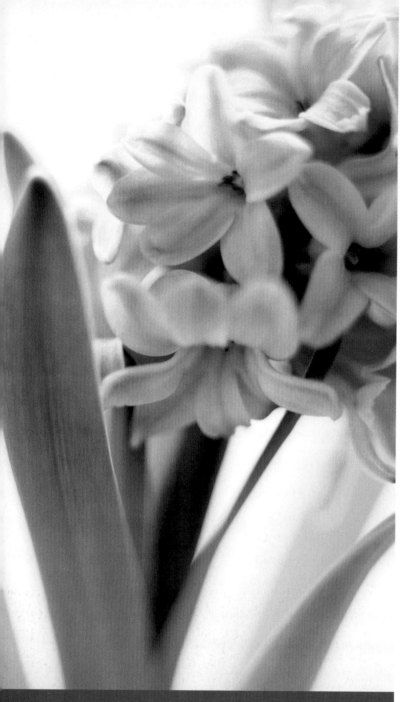

mantra

This is a powerful yet peaceful word, statement, or affirmation that you repeat over and over. Mantras are not limited to meditation. You can have a motivational mantra that you repeat to yourself when you wake up in the morning, or a calming mantra that you silently chant when you get stressed.

morning glow

There's another type of meditation I practice, but I'm not sure if *meditation* is the right word. It's this mental exercise I do in the morning when I wake up. I'm one of those rare people who actually enjoys waking up. I think that if you fall into that "let me sleep for five more minutes" cycle over and over then bolt out of bed at the last possible second and hop in the shower, you're missing a really beautiful moment of the day. Instead of lying in bed and hitting the snooze button a million times, enjoy that time when you're awake but not yet ready to open your eyes. Your consciousness is just coming to, your alpha waves are flowing, and you're departing your dream state.

These are some other great ways to start the day:

- Say thank you for the things that you have. You can thank a particular person or God, or you can just send thanks to the universe in general. Be grateful for your friends, family, health, job, the experiences you've had, even the bed you're in.
- Repeat an affirmation or mantra about the day ahead. Tell yourself you're going to have a great day, you're going to be energized, you're going to be safe, and you're going to have fun. Anything you want to emphasize is fine.

These little things can really affect your day in a beneficial way. Of course, I still punch the snooze button from time to time, but once you train yourself to have that moment, it becomes easier to wake up and face the world.

attitude on gratitude

Gratitude is one of my favorite words. There are so many things that you and I should be thankful for, yet we only focus on the things we're unhappy with, or the things we don't have. Take some time each day and remind yourself of what you do have. This is great to do when you're stressed out. Even if your job makes you crazy, be thankful that you have a job because a lot of people don't.

I know there will be times when you don't feel grateful for anything, but try thinking about this: Someone's always going to have it better than you and someone's always going to have it worse. That's the funny thing about life. The key is being thankful that you're not the latter and to stop comparing yourself to the person who you think has it better.

Gratitude is a great tool because it releases us from a negative cycle of thinking. Once we break free, there's a real possibility of change.

the golden rule
We all know it. Do unto others as you would have others do unto you. Pretty wise words. Don't get me wrong. I often have to remind myself to do the right thing. It's rarely our automatic impulse to take the high road, but you'll be amazed how good you feel when you do. Here are a few things to try:

stop gossiping. Gossip is all about negative energy and turns you into a petty person. Respect yourself enough to rise above judgment and gossip. Try to be the best person you know how to be and assume that those around you are doing the same thing. Remember that being a forgiving person is an act of gracious beauty.

donate something. Give a dollar to a homeless person. You don't know the circumstances he or she is facing. Send a check to a charity you believe in. Even five dollars can make a difference. You also can donate your time. Have you ever considered volunteering? There's no better way to feel good about yourself, share your gifts, and give back to the world around you.

send someone a card for no reason. No one sends letters anymore. Imagine how nice it would be to collect your mail and find an unexpected "thinking about you" card tucked inside a pile of bills.

say hello to a stranger. Once a day, pick someone nice and pleasant-looking (no stalker types)

kyanism

Think Positive Have you ever heard the term "creative visualization"? How about "the power of positive thinking"? Anytime you hold a certain thought in your brain, you legitimize it, whether it's good or bad. We rarely dwell on the good things; instead, we all have a strong tendency to obsess over the bad things. The thing is, whenever we spend time worrying or freaking out about something, we're actually meditating on it. If you make use of your ability to switch your brain in a different direction, you can turn worry into simple contemplation. Instead of visualizing the worst-case scenario, picture the positive outcome. If you're stumped by a certain problem, daydream about the possible solutions. Actually walk through them in your head like they're a mini-play with all the appropriate characters, scenery, and dialogue.

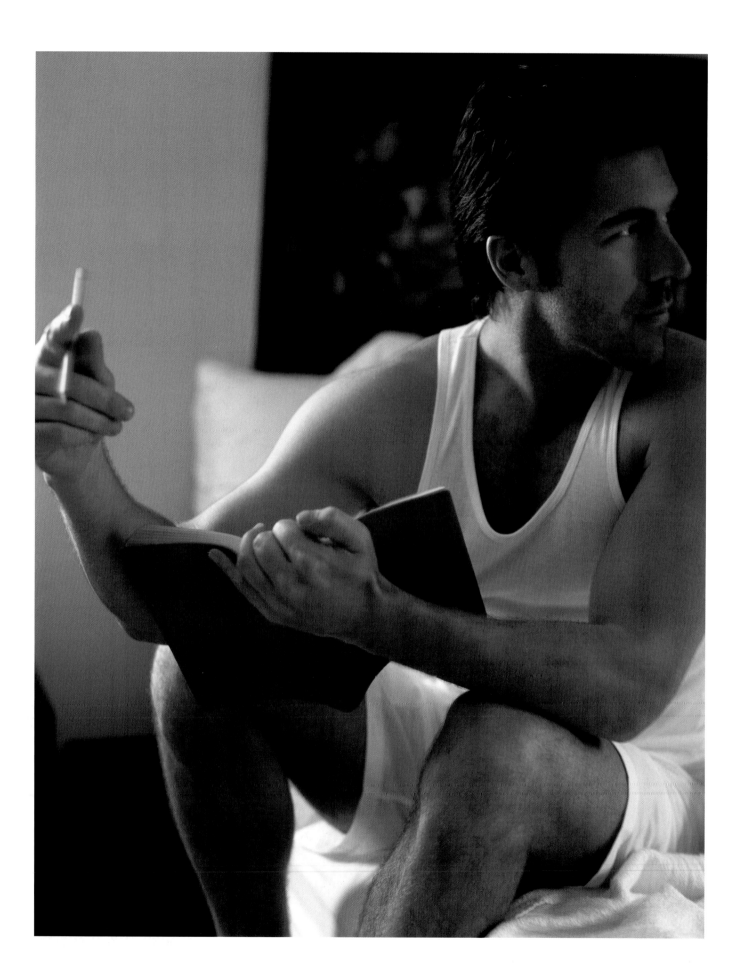

and say hi, good morning, good afternoon. Don't worry if they don't say it back. They're probably not used to being acknowledged.

mind your manners. There's a lot to be said for good manners. Opening a door for someone, giving up your seat to someone who's pregnant, and helping your neighbor with her groceries are considerate things. When you practice good manners, it often inspires others to get their behavior in line.

dear diary Keeping a journal is another form of meditation and positive thinking, and it's an amazing way to get yourself and your thoughts in order. Before you have an important meeting, a serious conversation with someone, or even a celebration, write down everything that's on your mind. List your anxieties, fears, hopes, expectations, and worries. Don't stress over punctuation or spelling. No one's going to see this except you. (Be smart about where you keep your journal. You don't want your private thoughts made public.) Once you've gotten everything off your chest, you can let it go.

Use your journal for other exercises. Record the different experiences and emotions you have. Fill it with lists of your dreams and goals, places you want to visit, things you want to do. Writing all of this down is another form of creative visualization.

life is not a beauty pageant Let this sink in for a moment. The irony of this book is that your value doesn't come from anything external. Sure, looking and feeling your best is important because it sends a powerful message to the rest of the world: "I care about myself." Once you believe that you are the best you can be physically—and I hope *Beautified* has given you the tools to feel this way—it frees you to focus on what's important. It's hard to concentrate on being a better person when you feel overweight or unattractive or second-rate, but now you have the power to change what you don't like. And you understand that sometimes the most important thing to change is not your looks but your mind-set.

Your beautification process never has to come to an end. Every morning is another chance to travel a little further on your journey. You might hit some roadblocks, or have to turn back a few times, but you'll make progress. Be open to that and you have the potential to improve upon something very, very beautiful: you.

kyanism

The Secret to Life

If anybody has the answers, it's the Dalai Lama, right? He was speaking in Central Park on my very first day of living in New York City (which I took as a very auspicious sign). I went to the park, along with thousands of other people, and struggled to hear what he had to say. He spoke for two hours and said some amazing things, but what really stuck with me were his final words: "Be nice."

credits

index